HOW TO IMPROVE YOUR SOCIAL SKILLS:

A GUIDEBOOK FOR ADULTS TO EFFECTIVE COMMUNICATION IN LOVE, WORK, LIFE OR ANYWHERE! 4 ESSENTIAL KEYS ABOUT LISTENING AND SPEAKING THROUGH TRAINING AND ACTIVITIES.

By reading this document, the reader agrees that under no circumstances is the author responsible for any losses, direct or indirect, which are incurred as a result of the use of information contained within this document, including, but not limited to, — errors, omissions, or inaccuracies.

I0499903

Description

Introduction

Conclusion

Description

Over the years, social agents have worked to making social skills better. Working on social skills takes time. Some people are just fast at learning while others are not. The fast people are natural at making conversation. The more one is able to make easy and relatable conversation then he or she forms bonds with others. The better the conversation then, the better the relationship. The relationships could be family, work relationship or even friendship.

The purpose of social skills is to develop conversations. Conversation skills are learned and nurtured over time. For one to be a good converse, then he or she must master confidence. Confidence is all that leads to a conversation. One must take a chance at others if he or she wants to make conversation. Well talking to others might come naturally while to others not so much. They then have to put in some effort and ensure that the conversation goes on without any hitches. After one has taken a chance on others, then one should talk the other people

The basic essential of conversing with people is one's ability to listen to them. It is always a good thing to listen to any situation. It is a bad habit just to talk and talk without listening. The people who keep and keep talking without listening to others are very annoying and are mostly ignored. One should learn to converse while listening to others. The conversation should not be one-sided, that is to avoid boredom. It is essential to know the art of talking while listening. The book has clearly shown the steps one must take to be a better listener.

This guide will focus on the following:

- The benefits of better conversation skills
- Enhancing social skills and social skills at work
- Overcoming lack of confidence and the fear of being judged
- Obstacles many of us face regarding charisma
- How to improve your listening skills
- How to attract and keep great friends
- Looking at things from a new angle
- Broaden your horizons
- Social/communication skills at job interviews
- Understand people emotions
- Keep a conversation going
- Identify your purpose
- Empathy... AND MORE!!!

Introduction

Development of better communication skills can be advantageous in various aspects of a person's life. It has the potential to help a person to develop a good professional career, good social reputation, and improve one related to his or her family. The current globe is hectic to get through things because of the over-reliance on the circulation of information. Social skills can be referred to as the skill set a person uses to help them relay information to people. These skills cut across what a person speaks, a gesture he or she uses, personal appearance and body language being used.

Social skills are supposed to be improved in the daily life of a human being. It has diverse benefits because human beings are social creatures. We are designed is a special way that we can communicate several things to people around us. The most communicated things by human beings are messages, thoughts, and feelings. A person's level of social skills is able to influence what is said by a person to the intended audience. There are two types of people when it comes to the level of social skills. There are people who are good social at interactions, and there are people who are poor at social interactions.

There are various advantages of having good social interactions in someone's life. These advantages are very distinct from each other. They include

- More and better relationships
- Great efficiency
- Better communication
- Advancement of a person's career
- Increased level of happiness

1. More and Better Relationships

People are able to identify themselves with individuals easily through this attribute. A person is able to be charismatic when he or she develops this trait. Charisma is one of the desirable traits in the current society. Several people are very interested in and attracted to charismatic individuals. The attraction goes beyond to also charismatic people being attracted to each other. This helps an individual create more relationships which are of good quality. It is very difficult for a person to advance in the world today without a strong level of personal relationships. Strong interpersonal relationships help a person to get promotions and employment through friends and families. This helps a person to have a well-honed social life with fewer amounts of stress.

2. Greater Efficiency

A person can easily avoid people he or she does not want to be around if he or she is good with people. There are people who tend to fear social interactions because people do not want to associate are available. These people who are not needed to be associated with may have different ways of viewing things or have different interests. There are situations in life where it is difficult to know who a person is meeting in several interaction points. The interactions might be offices, parties, or sacred places. However, a person who has good social skillset is much advantaged in such situations where he or she meets a person he or she is not interested in. He or she can easily socialize with other people in the congregation and avoid being lonely.

3. Better Communication

It is very advantageous for an individual to know how to relate to people both while alone or in groups. The process is very critical since it develops a person's communication skills. It is very difficult for an individual to have good social skills with a poor set of conversation skills. One of the most important skill sets a person can have in the information flooded era is being able to convey his or her information. The process helps a person be a better communicator in turn.

4. Advancement of a Person's Career

Having good social skill set cuts across people careers and how they succeed in them. Most of the lucrative career positions the current globe has an element of the social component. A deep and keener look in these posts involves a person having high levels of interaction with people. The common groups of people that persons in top positions interact with include media, colleagues, and employees. It is very difficult for a person to excel in a career when his or her office is isolated. Many organizations in the current employment market have also improved how they recruit employees. The organizations tend to look at a particular skill set that is tactical. An employee is supposed to have the ability to work with a team. He or she is supposed to be able to go to the extent of motivating and influencing his or her colleagues to be able to achieve organizational goals.

5. Increased Level of Happiness

The ability of a person to get along and being able to understand other people have the ability to improve a person's happiness in various ways. The various forms of happiness are generated from two sets of life which are personal or career happiness. People who are confident in workplaces have the potential of starting a conversation at workplaces or while in conferences. The idea can be a door opener to rise of rank, salary increase, or a new form of employment if they are ideally catchy. The personal side comes when a person is out of the official duties.

A simple smile and good articulation of greeting are able to make a person in social life. This acts as a spark to the formation of new relations to people around him or her. Creation of new relationships helps to play a very important role in a person's life. He or she is able to find a solid means of expressing him or herself. This is one of the good ways an individual has to reduce stress levels in his or her life through sharing or other bonding activities. A person is able to boost his or her self-esteem with the help of other people. Success from the two sets of life improves a person's levels of happiness and satisfaction. In turn, a person is able to have a good outlook in life.

Chapter 1 The Benefits of Better Conversation Skills

Having top-notch conversation skills is very vital in a human being daily lifestyle. Conversations held by an individual are supposed to swift in the modern age. This is irrespective of which massage, feeling, or idea is passed to an intended party.

Conversation can be described as the process which entails sharing and understanding the meaning. Successful communication entails two critical things which are to understand and be able to be understood. There is the process of successful communication is achieved through several ways which include;

- Verbally; this is the use of a person's voice.
- Written; the written form includes the use of books and mails
- Visually; it is the use of images, maps, and graphs.
- Non-verbally; use of body language, gesture, and eye contacts are applied in this case.

Listening is a very critical component of having a successful conversation. People in society often overlook the idea. It is because these set of people are more focused on what they say rather than what is been told to them by other people. A great person is able to be distinguished in people by his or her ability to pause and listen to others. It always portrays the virtue of respect and willingness from the other party in listening to those around him or her. Active listening skills and will help a person in developing good communication skills.

There are myriad importances of having better skills of conversing which are;

- Being valued in the place of work
- In demand by business
- Helps to improve a person's career
- Helps a person to speak concisely
- Assists in building better rapport with clients
- Influences the learning process
- Helps to create a better professional image

Six Importance of Having Better Skills of Conversing

1. Being Valued at the Place of Work

A person is supposed to demonstrate a certain level of communication skills while applying for a new job or seeking promotion. The high-class level of communication that can steer an individual to have this success include the ability to speak with several kinds of people from different backgrounds while maintaining good eye contact and use of fluency in the language used in communication. The ideas presented by a person are supposed to be appropriate when presented even in the form of writing. This helps a person get an advantage because he or she can work with a group.

An individual who is able to put people at ease, able to listen to them and speak clearly to them, is a very valuable person in an organization. This involves a demonstration of various skills such as;

I. Being able to listen and show interest in what people say
II. Having an appropriate manner in dealing with telephone conversations
III. Ability to persuade people
IV. Asking questions or expressing opinions clearly
V. Encouraging the team, a person is in

2. In Demand by Business

Both written and oral communication proficiencies have been ranked consistently across the employment market as the top ten skills that are desirable by employees. Various employees across the world are advised to take courses that offer a chance in the improvement of communication skills. These courses can either be online trained or in-person trained. The most common skills looked at by employers are communication skills, the ability of one to be organized, team working, analytical thinking, and critical thinking.

3. Helps in Improvement of One's Career

A person will be required to seek information, discuss issues, give out orders, work in teams, and interact with people at work. A person with good communication skills is able to undertake these activities with ease. It is because communications prove to a lubricant in enhancing cooperation and cooperation in organizations. The global community has been narrowed because of technology making the issue become of global attention.

Therefore, being able to be understood and understand others has positive effects on a person and a company he or she works for. This can help elevate a person to different ranks up to the international level. Employees want workers who can think about their own, find solutions to problems, and invent things with the help of people around them. It is not about doing a task well since other factors can elevate a firm.

4. Helps a Person to Speak Concisely

It is normal for people to feel nervous when he or she is talking to a person who is a higher rank than him or her. However, a person with good communication skills has the potential of knowing how to communicate best in any situation presented to him or her. The skill is essential at this point because it helps a person get the best out of a slippery position.

5. Assists in Building Better Rapport with Clients

Clients have one important desire than is always at heart. This group of people seeks to be understood by companies or firms because it helps them feel like they are valued. This feeling is achieved when they are contented, they have been heard and listened to. There are certain points employees in an organization interact with clients; successful firms are always formed by these moments since they keep client needs first after listening to them.

6. 6. Influences Learning Process

Communication skills highly influence the processes of imparting knowledge and believe. The learning process involves publicly speaking, and the answering question posed and airing out one's opinion. The process also involves writing; however; a person learns how to read first then he or she is taught how to write. Presence of good communication skills helps a person to grasp information and air out his or her opinion is clearly.

7. Helps to Create a Better Professional Image

Having good communication skills helps a person to build a good first impression. People in the current work are so obsessed with conveying a positive image as their reflection when they first meet with people. This is very critical in the business world because it portrays one's company or business. A person's professionalism while handling people at the first meeting is critical for business success in deals.

Chapter 2 Enhancing Social Skills And Social Skills At Work

The importance of good social skills cannot be overemphasized. It is a vital part of being human and being able to cope with others. It is a vital ingredient that can set you up for success in your career, relationships, and can also determine the level and quality of relationship you have.

The thought of striking a conversation with a stranger or asking a beautiful girl out sends a cold chill down the spine of many. The good news, however, is that you can take a step to build and improve your social skills. This chapter will be shedding light on simple and effective tactic you can use to get your social skills in order. Even if you are an introvert, applying these tips can make you appear confident and get along with everyone.

Some tested tips for improving your social skills are discussed below:

Talk a Little More than You do

We are talking about being social here right, and it involves talking! We understand it might be asking a lot that is why the recommendation is for you to talk a little more than usual. Do not just stop at "hi" and "How are you?" To make friends with those around you, you need to really show interest in knowing them. And the best way to do this is by talking.

We understand that small talk can be uncomfortable for socially awkward people. The idea is not to push yourself overboard, rather, we recommend putting a few more sentences out there. As a result of this, you need to get comfortable asking open-ended questions and avoid giving a yes or no answer.

Make sure you practice this at every opportunity you get. It could be at the grocery store or on the bus. It does not have to be an elaborate conversation. It is simply a call to add in a few sentences to express yourself.

This exercise is vital to improve your social skills because putting a restraint on expressing yourself will make you lose the social acuteness important in a social setting to keep people's interest. In other words, when you assume people are not interested in what you have to say, you kill every opportunity and avenue to mingle.

Offer a Simple Compliment

This is one of the simplest things you can do to enhance your social skills. The reward is high, with no risk in any form. As a matter of fact, people tend to flow toward and appreciate whoever makes them feel good. In approaching other people, what do you fear most? It is typical of people to assume they will make a fool of themselves they will stutter or come off as a bother.

I am not here to give you false hope that your assumption is baseless. My aim is to offer you the antidote which is to say something nice to people, someone, anyone! It does not have to be someone you know, and it could be the girl you always have an eye on, a coworker, male or female, in a group setting, in a train or a bus, anywhere. The idea is to shower many people with compliments and make them feel good. Some samples are:

- Cool watch!

- You have a terrific smile

- I love your smile

- What a neat shirt!

- You are so charming

- What lovely hair

Be sure to make eye contact as you smile. It is very important as you dish out this dose of compliments. It is not about whispering it as you sprint past them. Why is this foolproof? There is zero chance that you can be shut down since you are not putting out a request that can be shut down.

Besides, who does not like it when people notice and say good things about them? When you do this, and accompany it with a smile, there is no way it will not yield good fruit. You have succeeded in catching them off guard in a pleasant way. I bet you, either of two things will happen. Either they respond with a sincere thank you or stand there bedazzled that someone cared enough to notice a good thing about them.

And lastly, since you are not making any requests whatsoever, it is pretty rare that you will be blown off. How awesome it is to be that kind stranger who went out of his comfort zone to make someone else's day!

As a hint, older women, especially those above the age of fifty, respond positively to compliments from everyone. This is a good place to start then as you build your confidence, feel free to progress to the average person on the train. With time, the nervousness will die down and you get better at it. Bear in mind that there is at least one person who will appreciate your compliment and continue the conversation. This is progress!

Compliment Plus a Simple Question

I believe by now you agree that dishing out compliments to people comes with no harm in any form. Once you have mastered this, it is time to spice it up a little.

If you want to move past just dishing out compliments, you can graduate to adding a simple question. Since your question was accomplished with a compliment, there is little chance the person will shun you off. Here are a couple of examples:

- Your dog is so cute, what is her name?

- You cat is so lively! Where did you get them from?

- Your teeth are so white, what is your secret?

- Nice boots, where are they from?

Make Yourself Approachable

There are many elements that make up being approachable. We will, however, discuss two critical things that affect how easy it is to approach you. These are body language and facial expression. Bear in mind that people are constantly forming an opinion about others, and these opinions are based on the signal that they pick from you. In other words, people are deciding whether you are approachable without giving you the chance to defend yourself. This is why you have got to pay attention to your body language and facial expression.

What is Your Body Language Saying?

The way you carry your body is constantly sending messages to people. This is why you need to be mindful of the kind of vibe you are giving off through your body language. Folding your hands or crossing your legs, for instance, is a clear sign that you are closed to the conversation or interaction. This is a clear sign that indicates you are not interested in letting another person in. Giving out a slouched posture as well is like requesting that people should not notice you.

Since the way you carry yourself sends tons of messages, you can use this to your advantage. You can project a warm and open body language and hope that people get the message. This calls for a relaxed and open posture. Let your hands and legs be free. Do not lean against the wall or give a slouched posture, Stand straight and be part of the interaction. This will not make you closed off from the others.

What About Your Facial Expressions?

You cannot be making odd and funny faces and expect to get positive attention from people. People will most likely try to predict how you feel by reading your face. Your face is one of the factors that determine people's first impression of you. Wear a smile as often as possible. We are not asking you to be a clown, but be approachable with your smile. Laugh when someone says something funny and even if everything is not going on great, desist from letting it reflect in your face. If you are fond of wearing a straight face and rolling eyes at people, think of the kind of message it exudes. I bet you are not surprised at why you struggle at achieving social success.

Improve Your Conversational Skills

Being a good conversationalist is way different from being vast and able to speak confidently on many subjects. In trying to improve your conversation skills, let this sink into you that a good conversation involves two parties: a speaker and a listener.

And contrary to what you might assume, being a good conversationalist does not relate to your ability to talk much.

There is an aspect of active listening. This is a skill on its own, which involves paying attention to the conversation and giving cues to indicate that you are following as the conversation proceeds. For a conversation to be effective, it is important to give out signs that you are following it, and that the conversation is impactful. Even if the speaker does not say it, they are constantly looking for such signs from you, as this is a boost they need to communicate effortlessly. Example of such a sign is nodding, making eye contact, asking a question or even repeating a point that has been made.

You should also make an effort to keep the conversation flowing. One way to achieve this is by asking an open-ended question. These are questions that do not require a yes or no answer. Such questions will make the speaker elaborate more. For instance:

- What do you mean when you said that...?

- What do you think of....?

- Is that the only way to...?

The above is to give you a blueprint of how to keep the conversation going. The good news is that none of the above will give a yes or no response. This will prompt the conversation to flow naturally, giving you the insight to reduce anxiety and improve your conversation skills.

On a final note, it is also vital that you can contribute meaningfully to a conversation. People will value you if you can formulate and share your thoughts and arguments on the matter, rather simply nodding and giving an occasional yes.

Social Skills at Work

People are everywhere, especially in your workplace. Except you run a one-person business, you will need the services of others in your workplace. Even if you do, there are circumstances where you will need the input of others. In every phase of life, where you interact with people, you need social skills. It is one of the factors that can determine your success in the workplace. The good news is that social skills at work can be learned, and that is the aim of this section. If you find out that you are not getting along with people well, it might be that your social skills are lacking.

At work, you will meet various calibers of people, people of various backgrounds, upbringing, and attitude. It is with strong social skills that you will be able to relate with these categories of people. To develop the right relationship with your customers, co-workers, managers, and even juniors, your social skills need to be top-notch. Having explained how important social skills at work is, here are various ways you can them so you have an edge at your work

Managing Relationships

If you are a full-time worker, you will spend an average of eight hours each day at your workplace. That is one third of the hours you have in a day. If you spend this much time with people at work, it shows how vital it is to have and maintain a good relationship with coworkers. With a good relationship, you can get along with everyone, reduce conflict, and improve productivity.

Confrontation might not be the best way to solve a difficult situation at work. Maintain professionalism and politeness, and whatever you want to do, do it thoughtfully.

Empathy

One of the characteristics that will set you apart from others is the ability to understand other people's feelings. You need to listen and relate to other people's concern for you to have an idea of how they feel. This can guide you into helping people proffer solution to their problem since you know and understand what they feel.

Showing Cooperation

In any organization you find yourself within, I believe the firm will have the main goal. Besides, the main purpose of bringing a diverse group of individuals together is to help see such goal to fruition. This is why teamwork is one of the vital skills employers look for before hiring a candidate. Even with various individual task and different job description, the overall goal is the same. This is one of the reasons why you have to develop yourself to relate and work well with others.

It is the positive collaboration of the people in the company that will make it successful. As a result, people should be clear about their roles and what is expected of them. Make sure you encourage collaboration between coworkers and team members even if you are not the team leader. It is an attribute that will speak for you, if not now, in the future.

Showing Respect

There is this cliché that respect is reciprocal. If you want people to respect you, you have to show them respect. By respect, we mean being polite, mindful of your manners, being mindful of people's feelings, displaying good etiquette, and of course being mindful of how you address others.

Besides the points listed above, there are other ways you can show respect. Be sure to not interrupt people, or if you do, apologize for it and do not make a habit of it. Being a good, active listener is one of the most important ways you can show someone you value them and respect them. Even if you disagree with another coworker's opinion, do it respectfully. Be sure to listen actively while having a conversation and try not to interrupt. These simple skills go a long way in determining your success.

Be Mindful of Your Body Language

When it comes to social skills, the importance of body language cannot be overemphasized. This is why a whole section will be dedicated to body language in the later course of this book. From my research into body language, I have discovered that a person's body language can heavily contradict their words or the message they are trying to convey. In other words, even if they say one thing, their body is relaying a totally opposite message. As a result, it is not always about what you say, but how you say it.

In the workplace, be sure to always maintain an open and friendly body language, the type that is approachable. You cannot be carrying a stern face around and expect people to relate freely with you.

Speak Clearly, Confidently and in an Acceptable Tone

In building social skills at work, you want to appear confident. This calls for speaking clearly when you are engaged in any conversation. It is not about speaking very fast. Confident people pick their words without the pressure to speak fast.

In addition to speaking clearly, you also want to make sure you are using the right tone. Excessive loud tone can end up distracting everyone around, especially if it is an open workspace. We recommend taking note of how your coworkers communicate.

Join in Office Discussions

I am pretty sure you are not expected to work for eight or nine hours straight at work. There will be time for chitchats, lunch, and various other office discussions. It could be chats on entertainment like soccer or the latest movie, politics, etc.

Be confident enough to take part in such a conversation. Should an argument arise, be confident enough to present your points logically while respecting other people's opinion. And when other people's point is justified, against your view, be mature enough to acknowledge that you are wrong.

Practice Active Listening

There are many parts to active listening. It goes beyond allowing the words someone speaks to enter your ears alone. It involves giving complete attention and focus, with your body language all pointing to the fact that you are paying attention to what this individual is tell you.

Active listening involves putting forward a body language that shows that your attention is with the person. This calls for doing away with your mobile phone, computer, and pen. Not only is it a good way to show respect, but it also helps you understand the message being passed across better.

There is a Thin Line Between being Assertive and Aggressive

Everyone is entitled to their opinion, and everyone cannot have the same opinion on a subject. Even at that, sharing what you feel about a subject is not a crime, even if it means disagreeing with others. However, you have to be mature enough not to make others feel bad or stupid for sharing an opinion different from yours.

The ability to disagree and yet remain professional is an attribute you need to have.

In Conclusion

Without a doubt, it is important to pass here that without adequate social skills, you cannot survive in the workplace. Besides, even if you manage to survive, it can determine how far you go and your success. People who get what they want and get on the good side of their boss, have good social skills as one of the main factors that made this possible.

The good news is that you can take steps to work on your social skills. With some training and practice, you can take the necessary steps to develop your social skills in the professional setting.

Chapter 3 Overcoming Lack Of Confidence And The Fear Of Being Judged

If there is one thing that hampers the process of effective communication and prevents us from being our natural, confident and self-assured selves, it is an ever-looming fear of being judged by others. This is especially true of people who are shy or suffer from varying levels of social anxiety. They are perpetually functioning with a mindset that each time they speak or perform any action; the other person/people are judging them or secretly mocking them. The need to avoid leaving behind a negative impression is so compelling that they stop interacting with people altogether.

People can put themselves through highly self-defeating behavior to avoid the possibility of being judged negatively by other people. For starters, you may elude telling others what you truly desire to tell them. You may avoid speaking at work, parties or class for fear of 'not being good enough' or ridiculed. You may not tell your loved one your real desires, or you may hesitate to ask your manager for a raise. You may not want to tell a new date where you prefer to take them for dinner. The hesitation is arising as a result of fearing other people's judgment can impact all areas of your life and prevent you from enjoying more rewarding relationships by sharing authentic/genuine ideas, feelings, viewpoints, and emotions. You'll stop being yourself and try to be someone you are not just to please the other person or to avoid being judged by them.

The fear of judgment is deeply connected with the inherent need to be liked and accepted all the time. This can be psychologically rooted in our childhood and early adolescent experience. The need to be liked and accepted by others is so powerful that it stops us from communicating in an uninhibited manner. Thus, we are unable to express our true selves in the process. It is a fact that human beings are forever judging each other. They are always forming impressions about whether they like or dislike something or whether something is good or bad. Then, there are plenty of layers in between the two extremes. As we keep processing new information, our mind is assessing and reassessing things, which is a continuous process.

Rather than avoiding an issue by not mentioning anything about our opinions, feelings or preferences, and working in the direction of pleasing everyone all the time, try to overcome your own fear of being judged by people. Accept that the fear exists, and actively work on this fear or anxiety to tackle the bull by its horns.

Owing to this fear, they are unable to make meaningful conversations, engage in healthy discussions and enjoy fulfilling relationships with people. Are you someone who finds it excruciatingly painful to communicate with people for fear of being judged by others? If yes, you aren't alone. Here are some tips on overcoming this fear to facilitate more open, effective and fearless communication.

Judgments are unavoidable

Even the best and most successful people in the world are judged. Therefore, there is no escaping it. Resist the urge to control or influence other people's judgment about you. It will affect the way you communicate with them. There is only so much you can do to control other people's judgment about you. Don't demand that other people shouldn't judge you. It doesn't help to expect that we should be able to live without being judged unless you live in a rabbit hole. People have a tendency to judge other people words, actions, decisions, values, behavior patterns, beliefs, attitude, and ideologies. They may or not may express it, but they'll judge. It is a more physiological human brain process, where we take in information and process it using our own filters of biases, attitudes, beliefs, ideologies, prejudices and so on. It is almost an uncontrollable and involuntary process.

While communicating, make it easier for people to avoid judging you by sharing the context of your feelings. This will make it easier for people you are sharing the information with to understand you with the required understanding and compassion. Compassion is the ultimate judgment killer. Think of it is judgment's very own kryptonite. The two can rarely coexist. When compassion, understanding, and sensitivity are around, judgments have little power. Context offers people the opportunity to understand your situation with greater empathy by placing themselves in your shoes. Thus, there is no tendency to judge you.

For instance, if you are telling someone that your relationship is almost ruined because your partner is constantly at the receiving end of your suspicions, also offer some background information or context to help them view things from your perspective. In the above example, the listener is likely to judge you as an over possessive, jealous or suspicious partner. However, if you mention that you've been cheated and lied to in past relationships, which feeds your fear of being cheated in the current relationship, the person may understand you more effectively. Give people enough information to help them see things from your perspective and avoid making sweeping judgments based on stray facts here and there.

Bring about a shift in your perception

One way to beat the fear of being judged is to bring about a clear shift in your perspective in the company of other people. Divert focus on another aspect instead of emphasizing on what and how other people are thinking about you. Try to focus on conversations while also attempting to be in sync with other people. Understand that much as you'd like to focus on who or what you are, people do not focus on it.

Even if you say something awkward or your actions are embarrassing in your opinion, people barely notice them. We may obsess about a small thing we may have said to someone weeks ago, and unrealistically expect that the person is still holding on to it pretty much like us. There are high chances the individual has completely forgotten about it and moved on to other things. Their memories aren't as powerful as you imagine it to be.

During the process of communicating with people, if you experience the fear of being judged by others, find something to focus on soon. A majority of times, the fear of being judged isn't as apparent to the other person as we think. Focus on some sensory experiences connected to the event to shift attention from what the other person is thinking about you or how he/she is judging you. How do your surroundings look, smell and feel? What type of sounds do you hear? Is there music playing in the background? How does the food being served taste? This is especially true in social situations where we are always anxious about being misjudged by people, we are meeting for the first time.

This will help divert your attention from the fear symptoms to having a good time by interacting in a friendly and meaningful manner with the other person. Let's us assume you are a corporate networking event. Here, everyone is nervous about making a favorable first impression. Similarly, during a recruitment interview, all potential candidates are jittery about making a favorable first impression and eventually being hired by the organization.

Understand that irrespective of the situation you are in, almost everyone is sailing in one boat. This makes it easier for you to deal with your fear of being judged in certain situations.

Identify your strengths and weaknesses

When you know your inherent strengths or are confident about what you are great at, you are less likely to bother about what others think about you. The tendency to be affected by other people's judgments is far less when we are confident and aware of our own capabilities. Be self-assured about your strengths and know your shortcomings better than others. If someone forms an opinion or judgment about you, they are forming that judgment based on their filters, which may not have much to do with your own abilities.

When you are aware of your abilities or strengths, other people's judgments will wield less of an impact on your during the process of communication. While talking to people, be aware of your own strengths, personality characteristics, and vulnerabilities. This way, the impression others form about you will not hold much relevance for you. You will continue saying what you have to in staying true with your own nature. Do not allow others to kill your individuality, personality, and character based on their judgments about you.

When you don't believe in or stand for something, you will tend to believe everything. Similarly, when you don't have a clear understanding of your own personality, strengths, and attributes, you will believe whatever others think about you. Lack of confidence or self-awareness is the biggest catalyst for being affected by other people's judgments. Take stock of your own strengths and weaknesses while communicating with people to avoid going with whatever they want you to believe about yourself. Assume charge of how you view yourself if you want others to view you positively.

Everything is temporary

You will rarely fear judgments if you realize that nothing about these judgments or what people think about is permanent. The thing about the human brain is, it has the capacity to process limited data. Though we make innumerable judgments, they don't' have a place in the memory bank forever. However, much you believe otherwise, people are not going to remember that one awkward moment of yours forever or every time they meet you. There is only so much information one can practically retain in the realms of the brain and conscious memory.

When people make certain judgments or impressions about, there are high chances that a few days or even moments later that judgment may have left their conscious awareness. Our understanding of people is not made based on the tiny setbacks, awkwardness or mistakes in what they say or do. For all you know that one moment you thought you were really awkward and people will remember it for a lifetime, they may forget about it before saying goodbye to you after the first meeting.

Though an overall impression about people is quickly formed when we meet them (remember the first four seconds rule?), our understanding of others is not based on their minor behavior patterns or words. It is more dependent on a pattern of the schema of big things that others say and do. There is a pattern in the manner with which they interact with us and make us feel over a period of time. This is how we form an impression or judgment about them. If the overall pattern of your words, actions, and behavior with other people are positive and favorable, they will not form negative judgments about you based on one stray moment, a wrong word used here and there or an awkward action.

The human brain considers a larger perspective in a broader schema of things. Thus judgments, opinions, and perspectives change over a period of time. It isn't now and never; however scary it may appear to be. You may not have a second chance to make a first impression, but during the course of your interaction with the person, you do have an opportunity to establish a pattern.

You are not being judged all the while

Keep in mind that this looming fear of being judged by people every time exists in your mind and isn't real. This is a more extreme and unrealistic type of thinking that leads us to believe that we are being judged all the time. A more balanced and real perspective is – no one really gives a damn! Honestly, people are more preoccupied (especially if they are meeting you for the first time) with how other people perceive them than forming opinions about others. Believe it; people are as nervous about interacting with you for the first time as you are. A majority of our social phobia or anxiety originates from the notion that we are being judged all the time. That's far from reality or rational thinking;

People have more on their plate then judging you. This fear of being held under the microscope for every word and action will prevent you from communicating with others in a meaningful and rewarding manner.

Bear in mind that others don't always make you the center of their focus during the process of communication. They are more often than not thinking about what to say or do next instead of forming an opinion about you. Even when people think about it, they rarely think about you in the manner in which you think about yourself. Try to analyze people's thoughts while communicating with them. What are they implying through their verbal and non-verbal communication patterns? They seldom perceive you in the same negative light that you perceive yourself. Take advantage of multiple social contexts to shift your negative or self-defeatist thoughts. Stop the cycle of negative thinking in its tracks by performing a physical action (thinking biting your tongue or pinching yourself) to snap yourself out of the thought process.

Once you realize your negative thinking is impeding the process of communication, get back to communicating naturally and uninhibitedly with people. Adopt a more neutral communication process if you find it challenging to make it overtly positive.

Practice challenging your thoughts by thinking of evidence that is contrary to what you believe. Is there solid proof that you make a complete fool of yourself every time you talk or interact with people? Is there glaring evidence pointing to the direction that people don't like to talk to you or are disinterested in you every single time? Keep thinking on evidence to the contrary when you find yourself being bogged down by negative thoughts.

Bear in mind that to a certain extent, everyone is anxious while communicating, especially if they are meeting you for the first time. At some level, all people struggle with some fear or anxiety of being judged. Understanding this can help you realize that no one's judging, ridiculing or criticizing you all the time. They are in fact dealing with their own fears, uncertainties, and insecurities, far from being obsessed with judging, seizing you up or criticizing you at the level you imagine.

Beating the fear of being judged while communicating needs effort and practice and cannot be overcome in a single day! Develop new thoughts, behavior patterns, ideas, social skills, and more.

Preparation is the key

We are more confident, self-assured and in control of our words and actions when we know what we are doing. The more we prepare, the more confident we are while approaching and conversing with people. Keep all facts, figures, and numbers handy. Have genuine interest to understand people's desires, preferences, likes, interests and so on. Listen to them carefully to understand what the other person is trying to convey through both verbal and non-verbal communication.

Practice and preparation reduce your fear of being judged. One of the best ways to conquer your fear of being judged during the communication process is to observe how you appear and feel while communicating. What are your typical expressions, gestures, movements, posture and so on while talking to people? How do appear while interacting with other people in varied situations? Stand facing a mirror, and pretend to talk to people, address an audience or make a presentation. How do you look and feel? Do you feel more confident when you realize you don't appear as bad as you think you do? Does facing yourself in the mirror increase your confidence and sense of self-worth?

If you are going for an interview, practice answering in a perfectly calm, poised and confident manner. If you are approaching people at a business networking event, practice talking in a more approachable, open, welcoming and friendly way. Keep preparing and practicing multiple communication scenarios before the mirror until you no longer experience the fear of being judged. Even in the event that people come out guns and daggers after you, it may not take long for you to take them on in a more solid, confident and well-prepared manner. Being confident also awards you the strength to conquer the fear of being judged.

Keenly consider your own judgments

There's seldom a more effective way to stop being bothered by other people's judgments than to stop judging yourself and other people. At times, our fears are imaginary. People who suffer from social anxiety almost always believe that everyone is judging them. This fear is far from realistic or balanced. Watch your own thoughts, ideas, language and perception about yourself. What words do you use while describing yourself? How do you view your own words, actions, and behavior? Do you see your own actions or behavior patterns in a positive or negative light?

Obvious, sometimes judgments are unavoidable. If a person has been terribly rude or means to you, you aren't going to think they are angels incarnated. However, watch the words used in your head for certain people, behavior patterns and events. Reframe the focus on your own judgments. Rather than saying, "*someone sucks*" or "*someone is a total loser*", question yourself about the effect that person has over you, which you may want to avoid or gain awareness of in future.

For instance, "*He has never followed through with his commitments made to me*" or "*She tells me she's doing her best but ends up disappointing me*". Don't label people; instead, identify what they do to have a certain impact over you. Resist the urge to classify people as good or bad character. Instead, communicate in a manner that is healthy for you. If a certain behavior pattern on someone's part has an unhealthy effect on you, learn to identify its impact and deal with it instead of labeling people.

Watch the most common words you use for yourself. If you are constantly referring to yourself as "*loser*" or "*failure*", you are as guilty of judging yourself as others. The biggest barrier to the process of communication is our tendency to judge ourselves.

That little nagging voice in our head needs to be silenced more than anyone else. People will have countless opinions, notions, and ideas about you. They are entitled to their thoughts, and it isn't much you can do about it. This is an important step when it comes to overcoming the fear of being judged by people. If you are forever bogged down by what others are thinking about you during the process of communication, take stock of your own confidence, self-esteem, and sense of self-worth.

Identify how your inner critic addresses, and any negative thoughts that it ignites within you that hamper you from relating to other people. If your inner critic is constantly telling you that you are a fool when it comes to trusting people owing to a few bad experiences, you will not be able to trust people while conversing with them. Your beliefs and negative comments about yourself will lay the ground for your communication with other people, so watch what you say to yourself.

Know how much you contribute to the fear of being judged during the process of communication. What role does the filter of your own negative thoughts play when it comes to your fear of being judged? Take control of your actions, thoughts, and beliefs to start making small shifts in your perspective or thought process. Stay positive and optimistic instead of worrying about what others think about you.

Chapter 4 *Shyness*

Shyness refers to the tendency to feel nervous or timid when interacting with other people, especially strangers. Talking or engaging with people outside of your normal social circle can be frightening and you might find yourself avoiding these situations as much as possible.

If you think that you're struggling with shyness, welcome to the club. I mean even the most outgoing and socially competent person you know is struggling with some level of shyness. It's probably not going to be at the same level as you, it's probably not going to be that extreme but nobody is immune to this.

It's easy to see why this is the case because whenever you're out in public or you're dealing with other people, there is always a chance that you will fall flat on your face. That's right. There's always the risk that you will make a complete and total fool out of yourself.

That risk never goes away regardless of how good you become with people. That's just not going to happen. There is always that possibility, and at the back of your head, you're worried about it. Depending on how you deal with that, it can lead to serious problems or you can continue to do well.

Types of shyness

When people say that they're shy, they're basically making a blanket statement that doesn't really mean anything. I'm not saying that they don't feel certain things. I'm not saying that they are unclear as to what they're feeling. They're obviously feeling some sort of negative reaction to people. However, there are two kinds of shyness, and if you want to overcome it, you have to be clear as to what type of shyness you are struggling with.

1. Negative Association

The first type of shyness involves some sort of negative association. At some point in the past, you feel that you have made such a fool out of yourself in front of people who you equate or associate being in front of people with that negative feeling.

This negative association remains even though you are a better person now when it comes to social skills. That negative association remains despite the fact that now you are a better speaker.

That association is all in your head. You choose to keep it alive. You choose to continue to link being with people, going out in some sort of open social area with that negative experience.

2. Chemical Imbalance

The other type of shyness is harder to deal with because it's not just in your head. It's not just a simple matter of choice. Instead, there is an actual chemical imbalance in the neurotransmitter of your brain that triggers all sorts of negative physical effects. There are people who are so shy that they get physically sick.

I'm not talking about just feeling uneasy. I'm not talking about wanting to turn around because you are to just so afraid of what would happen. No, we're talking about actual physical symptoms. These people get sick to the point they vomit. They start trembling. In fact, a lot of people drop their knees and assume the fetal position and start rocking.

This is real stuff, and this is due to a chemical imbalance where finding yourself in any kind of open social setting where you're dealing with people triggers a negative chemical response. Your stress hormone levels shoot up, physical symptoms appear and you are trapped in a negative feedback loop.

It starts out with cold sweat. You're basically feeling clammy, and then you're feeling sweat forming and then you start behaving in a less optimal way.

People are not stupid. People can see this. So, they sit up and pay attention, your social performance suffers. They send you signals, and you interpret these in the worst way possible and your physical symptoms get worse and more.

What started out as simple cold sweat becomes buckets of sweat and then you start shaking and, before you know it, you want to throw up. In fact, before you know it, you want to physically turn around and run at full speed in the other direction.

The good news is that chemical imbalances can be fixed. You can't completely get rid of it just by using chemicals, but there are pharmaceutical products currently available that would help you deal with clinical anxiety disorder.

This is an actual clinical diagnosis. You need to see a psychiatrist to get the right medication. You also need to get counseling to lessen the symptoms.

However, you can fix this. This is not a death sentence to your social life. What I'm going to cover in the following sections deal primarily with negative associations because this is what most people suffer from.

Shy people are often victims of one simple Negative Association

It's easy to think that if you are very shy that you are essentially just harboring all these negative associations. You are under the impression that you have so many negative experiences in the past and these all combine together into this really oppressive feeling that you get when you're dealing with strangers, talking to people one-on-one or otherwise just being out there with other people.

What if I told you that is an illusion? What if I told you that there is really just one negative association that it all leads to? Everything else is just really a rehash of that one negative association.

You have to find this. You have to look at the negative experience that you suffered initially. This is what got the ball rolling. This is what triggered the whole sad situation.

The reason you're shy is that you equate being in any kind of social setting or participating in any kind of social activity with a negative experience. There's this unbreakable bond in your mind between the social setting or the social activity with a negative experience.

Now, what's wrong with this picture? You can engage in a social setting today, and there's no guarantee that negative experience will happen. In fact, usually, since you are a bit older, more experienced and more skilled, there's a good chance that the experience will be very positive. However, why do you hang on to this equation of social setting/activity = negative experience?

Break the Iron Link

Please understand that for you to overcome shyness, you have to break this link between a negative experience from the past and social activity now. Basically, what you're doing is you are saying to yourself that since I have a negative experience in the past due to social activity, this means that any social activity now and, in the future, will predictably result in a negative experience. That's too much of an assumption to make. Most people cannot tell the future.

Furthermore, like I said, you're better equipped now. You're a different person now. So, why beat yourself up unnecessarily by assuming that you will have a negative experience just because you were in some sort of social setting or engaged in a person-to-person social activity?

Break this iron link- Here's how you do it

The people around you did not cause the negative experience. Seriously. Sure, you might be thinking back and focusing on some people laughing, chuckling, pointing fingers, that of thing. However, let me tell you a lot of that stuff is just mental embellishment because the more you remember that negative or painful experience, the more you fill in details. If you're really honest with yourself in many ways, that did not happen, or you just basically blew things out of proportion.

Instead, the negativity can be traced to your reaction to that experience. You interpreted it in the worst way possible, you blew things up out of proportion and you just made things worse.

You need to change your reaction because if you continue to read that experience today, you continue to strengthen that bond or that link between social setting and activity and a negative experience.

Deprogram yourself

How do you deprogram yourself to get out from under this iron rink? I mean this is easy to say but hard to do. I can convince you that this is not a good thing, and you would absolutely, but that agreement is not going to do you much good because the moment a certain mental image flashes in your mind, you can't help but automatically respond in the worst way possible. All the old negative feelings come back over and over again.

Not surprisingly when you find yourself in a social setting, you start behaving the way you normally behave. You feel shy. You feel like you're being judged. You feel that something bad is about to happen. You feel awkward and on and on it goes.

You have to deprogram yourself. The first step to this is to understand that there are different ways to read "negative" social signals.

Remember: You are always in control

The bottom line here is actually pretty simple. Regardless of whether you're dealing with things from the past or things that are happening in front of you, you are always reading the situation. As the reader, you know you have a lot more control than you give yourself credit for. You read in meaning.

There is such a thing as subjective meaning. Yes, I admit that, but don't ever downplay the importance of subjective reading because things may not be as bad as you remember them. Things may not be as sad as you perceive them to be now.

Avoid the Negative Feedback loop

Given our power to read the worst into our daily activities, please understand that this really becomes almost irresistible because of negative feedback loops. We find ourselves in a situation where we end up reinforcing the very worst readings we can come up with of our daily stimuli. It doesn't have to be that way.

There is such a thing as a positive feedback loop. You can choose to flip the script. You can choose to create an upward spiral instead of a downward one. However, it is a choice.

Unfortunately, exercising that choice, knowing when to do it and how to do it requires effort and you watch repeated failures until you get good at it, but you have to do it. Otherwise, you end up with a negative feedback loop. This is how shyness becomes entrenched.

It becomes stronger and stronger because you feel that it is validated by reality. What you're really doing is you are just engaged in a negative feedback loop. You could have chosen differently. You could have flipped it around.

Here's how it normally works. You focus on your negative reading of the feedback.

For example, you see this really hot member of the opposite sex doing something seemingly directed at you. So, you give it the worst negative reading whatsoever. You interpret it as a complete and total condemnation, dismissal or rejection of who you are as a person. You feel completely unattractive, unwanted, unlovable, etc., etc.

You then feel shy because you don't want to be around other people because you feel that this is the kind of reaction you get. So, you perform badly. This can mean just running away from the social event, or this means going to and just nursing a beer, watching everybody else have a good time. Alternatively, if you at a dance club or an outdoor dance party, you're just dancing around in circles by yourself or with your narrow circle of friends.

This, unfortunately, draws more negative feedback. Well, at least you think they're negative. People will sit up and pay attention. You then interpret it the worst way again, the process repeats itself and you end up digging deeper and deeper into a negative emotional hole.

What do you think happens to your shyness in this context? It gets stronger and stronger. Basically, you're telling yourself, "This is objective proof that social settings are bad and causes me pain, makes me feel unloved, makes me feel unwanted and people can't accept me, there's something wrong with me" and on and on it goes.

There is good news here. You don't have to do it. You don't have to be stuck in that negative feedback loop.

Tips to Overcoming shyness

Shyness can indeed hold many people back because the shy ones tend to stay away from speaking up and public situations and somewhat because they always experience lasting anxiety. If you are one of those, keep calm and know that you aren't alone because 4 out of ten individuals consider themselves as being shy. However, here is the good part; you can overcome shyness with a will to change, effort and time, there is a possibility to succeed. If you have severe shyness, you may probably need a counsellor's or a therapist's help though most people are able to overcome the shyness by themselves.

Always keep it light

In a situation where people talk about your shyness, let your tone keep casual and if at all it turns out to be part of a conversation you are having, just talk of it cheerfully.

Do not tell

There is no need for you to tell about your shyness to anyone. The people around you know it already and there are others that can never even get the chance to notice. And it is not as noticeable as you may perhaps think.

Always avoid the label

Do not allow yourself to be described as shy. You are not a single trait but you are unique. Don't label yourself as shy or as anything else.

Avoid self-sabotaging

At times we tend to be our own enemy. Always analyze the power of that voice so that you can calm it. Do not allow your inner criticizer to bring you down.

Always pick your relationships cautiously

People who are shy tend to have few relationships but that are deeper which means that the choice of partner or friend is always more important. Always spend time with people who encourage you in your life and are warm and responsive.

Chapter 5 Obstacles Many Of Us Face Regarding Charisma

Of course, if being charismatic were easy, everyone would do it. Let's talk about the obstacles many of us face regarding our charisma, learned or otherwise.

The Importance of Knowing Our Worth

This can be a very challenging task, and it's not necessarily our fault if we're out of touch with our own personal sense of value. Perhaps we were raised by a care-giver who put us down, or lived with a sibling who constantly berated us. Maybe we had a long-term relationship with a partner who was toxic, and who whittled away our self-esteem. Whatever the reason for your flagging self-worth, understand that a) it's not your fault and b) it is your responsibility to do something about it. Healing can take a lot of time, but that's no reason to ignore the need for it. The best time to start something new is today, and right now.

A frequent topic of debate is whether it's true that "we can do anything". For instance, not everyone's capable of becoming a prima ballerina or a professional quarterback. However, if we zero in on this statement, and add some detail to it, it's actually true, if:

- We make sure that our bodies are capable of the task, and discover if there's help to assist us.

- We take the time to do the work necessary to accomplish the "thing", and
- Make sure the thing is something we truly want to do.

You might not ever break into professional American football, but you could turn out to be an excellent football coach at your local Boys and Girls club, or even play in an amateur league. You might not ever perform the Nutcracker at Radio City Music Hall, but you can certainly perform in local events, strengthen your body, and achieve your dream of becoming a dancer. Even those without the use of their legs have ran in marathons, played basketball, or performed in dance concerts. The key elements here are *focus, will, and determination.*

Now let's focus on you. What have you achieved that is still a source of satisfaction and pride to this day? If you've not yet achieved anything you feel is worthy of respect, what would you *like* to achieve? Also, go back and look at things you might not consider achievements, but with a positive eye. Perhaps you're downplaying yourself and masking real, impressive accomplishments.

There are statements you need to make, right now, in order to better yourself and put yourself in the charismatic mindset. These aren't promises—promises can be broken, especially if we're making them to ourselves. These are *statements*:

- I have the potential to achieve great things. I was born with this potential, and no one can take it away from me.
- I will not remain idle in my daily life. I will move forward and be a person of action.
- Following action, I will also give myself permission to rest, and relax. Both action and rest are necessary ingredients to success.
- I will not allow myself to pity myself. There's nothing to pity about me. I am okay.
- I will shift my focus from other people I used to think were better, to myself. I am good enough.
- I will dare to question myself, in order to make sure I'm authentic in my endeavors and behavior. Questioning does not mean hating. I refuse to engage in self-loathing.
- I am going to tap into my potential and achieve more with it.

Understand that you will never please everyone. If you believe that you can, you'll soon learn that trying to please everyone pleases no one, and ignores important care of yourself. Make peace with this and realize that not everyone is for everybody else. It's a wide world out there. You will find the people that you connect with.

Your opinions matter, and they also may change, and that is okay. Don't hide yourself for fear of being unpopular. At the same time, have the strength to *examine* your thoughts and opinions when you gain information and other people's points of view. It's okay to concede that you were wrong, or ignorant of something. Admitting that shows greatness, humility, and a mind that's not afraid to learn and grow.

Pleasing other people is not the point of the game. If it happens, great! If it doesn't, that's okay. Desperation is something that naturally drives others away from us; when we show this in our need to please others, we actually drive them away. When you're not afraid to displease or even offend others with your opinions, it shows strength and confidence. Don't *try* to offend, or take joy in offending others, because that's extremely unappealing, however, when you refuse to change what's vital and *true* about yourself to impress others, that in itself is incredibly impressive. You will make the right connections with the right people when you stand up for yourself with both strength and integrity.

Integrity is the name of the game, and having integrity shows that you don't consider human interaction a game. Other people are just as important as you are; no one should ever be placed above or below someone else. When you are capable of empathy and can put yourself in another's shoes, your words and actions will maintain integrity, and other people will find it easier to relate to you, as well as have respect for you.

What happens when your values change, and you make choices or take action that you would never have in the past? You can still maintain integrity. Integrity simply means that you act and speak in accordance with what you believe, and beliefs change as we mature. Integrity can and should be maintained throughout our lives. Never let fear, your own ennui, or other people's threats coerce you into being corrupted.

Our Inner "Weather" And How It Effects Our Outer Presence

Getting back to our "presence", when we find ourselves in social situations, what's going on inside our heads at the time greatly effects how others perceive us. Later on, in the book we'll discuss ways to cultivate happier mindsets and tackle charisma-killers such as anxiety, stress, and depression. Right now, let's focus on the immediate need for a clear, calm mind to project the best presence and maintain optimum charisma.

The nervousness you feel inside will be readily visible on the outside. Just like genuine joy, awkwardness is also contagious.

Refuse to feel shame. If you've made a mistake, it's perfectly acceptable and natural to feel regret regarding making that mistake. Then, using our determination (if the mistake only effected us) or our empathy (if it effected someone else) we can strive to correct that mistake, or at least ensure that it never happens again. In social situations however, shame should be left at the door. It doesn't serve us, and has no place in the charismatic person's repertoire or vocabulary.

What happens when you say something that offends someone? For starters, do not immediately apologize. Stand your ground, not with arrogance, but with quiet strength. Listen to the other person and strive to learn what about your statement was offensive. See if you can learn anything from that person's point of view, and be thankfully vocal about it if you do. Make statements such as "I see where you're coming from." Then, if the emotions have cooled and you've made every effort to understand the other person, you may choose to offer an apology—but make sure you can do that with honesty. Stop adding "I'm sorry" into every other moment of a conversation. It's neither genuine, nor attractive.

Lastly, if you haven't done this enough already, start practicing the art of thinking for yourself. Don't just go along with the crowd. Examine the information you're given with an open mind, but don't be gullible. Become your own person.

Social Awkwardness Explained

When it comes to social awkwardness, there is a lot of *bad* advice out there. For starters, it doesn't matter if "everyone" has felt socially awkward at one point or another—that's not going to help you, not one bit. It also doesn't help to tell you to just "snap out of it" or imagine everyone in the room naked.

I mean, that would be even more awkward, right?

The art of social fluency takes practice. The most common reason people are socially awkward is because they are simply not in enough social situations to have acquired any practice or skills. If you want to be charismatic, you're going to have to do the work; there are no shortcuts.

Spending more time with people, you're going to begin to develop a sense of conversational and social rhythm: when to speak, and when to listen; when to tell a joke and when to keep the topic serious. If you spend most of your time alone, there's no way you're going to achieve this kind of intuitive interactional skill set. Watching actors in conversation might be a start, but we're also not always seeing characters at their best, and most importantly, *we* are not in the conversation—we're only watching it on the screen.

Anything you're skilled at—usually, unless you have a particular knack or gift in that certain area—you will have started out with some degree of awkwardness. Driving a car, writing a resume, mastering a video game, shaving, curling your hair—*it all takes patience and practice.* So, resign yourself to the fact that if you want to be charismatic, you're going to need time, patience, and practice. Then approach this task with passion, because that will help too!

Muscle memory pertains to speaking, also. It also helps us with our facial expressions. We mimic each other all of the time, this is how babies learn to speak and express themselves, and this is how we learn to convey the emotions we feel—by watching other people. The more you work those muscles in a certain way to connect with a certain idea or emotion, the easier it will be, the more *natural* it will become, to express yourself with ease and grace in the future.

Social awkwardness comes when we don't exercise these muscles often enough. Spending too much time by ourselves can make these skills "rusty", or underdeveloped.

Determining Whether You're on the AS (Autism Spectrum), and Why It's Not a Bad Thing If You Are

Everyone in fifty-nine people in the world will be born with autism. Male children are more apt to be on the autism spectrum than women. What is autism? For starters, it's not necessarily a setback. While approximately one third of people on the spectrum have some amount of intellectual disability and/or are non-verbal, others, such as those with Asperberg's Syndrome, do not. (Pronounced asz-*PURGER'S)*. You see, autism is a *spectrum* of brain behavior and recognition. There are many different ways to be on the autism spectrum.

Asperger's is called a "high-functioning" placement of autism. One of the trademarks of having Asperger is having an acute interest bordering on obsession in a certain topic or topics. While this can be challenging during childhood (imagine an elementary school age kid trying to have in-depth discussions of World War II or cryptobiology and you'll get an idea), for adults, it can actually be quite an advantage. A kid obsessed with dinosaurs to the point of memorizing every bone of every species uncovered could have quite a career at a museum or professor of paleontology.

A trait that occurs in people with Asperger's is also a large vocabulary obtained at a young age. People with Asperger's may discover that they intimidate people with their knowledge and vocabulary, but ironically feel intimidated themselves by those people.

What's important to realize is that very often, people with Asperger's don't realize they have a "problem", generally speaking, until adulthood, and their behaviors and the way they look at the world is only labelled a problem by other people, or by themselves if they've been shamed for being awkward in social situations. People on the autism spectrum simply process the information that life gives them differently. That does not make them necessarily "stupid" or "weird". They often have mental and imagination-based gifts that people not on the spectrum do not possess.

However, having Asperger's can pre-dispose you to:

- Avoidance of eye contact (without even realizing it!). A classic sign is someone with Asperger's telling a story to someone, but looking past their shoulder or away while telling it, often making the listener ask, "What are you looking at?"
- Difficulty taking turns.
- Difficulty in making new friends.
- Being prone to conversations that revolve around yourself and your own interests.
- Occasionally, socially-inappropriate behavior. This usually stems from processing things differently, and often out of an attempt to be humorous in a social setting.
- Taking things literally and not understanding common social cues, such as high-fiving, or expressions like "sharp as a whip" to indicate intelligence.
- Some Aspie folks have heightened senses, such as the sense of smell, making those who wear too much cologne or perfume unbearable to be around.
- Finally, for someone with Asperger's, it may be difficult to express their impressions about things to non-AS people. Many people with Asperger's also have something called "synesthesia", where they see music in shades of colors, or can describe the flavor of something in number patterns or unusual choice of words. For these people, senses become combined or switched around.

Since there is a lot more awareness about the autism spectrum now, kids diagnosed early enough get special help at school, such as small classes where they meet once a day to go through "typical" social situations and learn good choices and responses that will keep them in the loop. And while becoming inauthentic to one's self is never a good idea, even to gain popularity, we all have social "tics" and quirks that can be worked through to make us engage with other people more comfortably and smoothy. People with Asperger's just sometimes need a bit more help in that area.

If you think you might have Asperger's, talking to your doctor or therapist, or taking an online test can help you determine whether the description fits you. Once knowing this about yourself, it can be easier zeroing in on the social skills you need to work on the most. Just remember, there is nothing shameful about being born on the autism spectrum. It's genetic, it's common, and people on the spectrum can live a full, vibrant, and fulfilling life.

If you are on the spectrum, or know that you have Asperger's, there are ways that you can get an edge on improving your social prowess. Begin by making a list of things that make you uncomfortable, socially. Separate them into these three categories:

- Things That Confuse Me (such as how to begin a conversation, tell a funny story)

- Things That Worry Me (such as the fact that you're not social enough, or what other people will think of you if you try to become more social)
- Excuses I Make To Avoid Being Social (such as taking on extra shifts at work, or binging an entire television series over a weekend)

Take a good, hard look at the things that worry you. If any of them sound silly, then that's a good thing! That means you're halfway towards eliminating them altogether. Underline or circle any of the worries that look less worrisome once you read them over.

Next, look at your excuses. Becoming more charismatic involves self-analyzing, and this is a challenging task for *everyone,* not just folks on the spectrum. Which of these excuses can be lessened (such as only watching three episodes per weekend of a show), and which would you be able to tackle first, so that over time, you slowly eliminate all of them?

Face your social fears, but do it slowly, one step at a time. There is no need to push yourself here—just *wanting* to get better at socializing is a step in the right direction. As long as you make steady progress, you will reach your goal.

Pay attention to when you try something new that landed on your list of "Worries". What happened when you tried it? How did everyone react? Chances are, it will not have been as bad, or not have been bad at all, as you first feared. Picture how you would react if you met someone who say, stumbled in their words or made an awkward joke. Would you have empathy for them, or would you ridicule them? Once you see that most people will opt to be kind in a social setting, it will be easier for you to reduce your fears in a realistic way.

Finally, if you exhibit any physical symptoms in social settings (or when you're preparing to go to one), such as feelings of panic, trouble breathing, sweating, increased heart rate or dizziness, consider talking to your doctor about trying anxiety medication or CBD. CBD is a non-narcotic derivate of the cannabis plant. It cannot make you feel "high" or intoxicated, but it has been proven to be an excellent tool in fighting anxiety and depression. Many people use it with good results, not just people with Asperger's.

Other steps to help in social settings include:

- Learning and understanding anything that's confusing to you. Reach out to a trusted family member or friend to discuss and even "practice" things that have baffled you in past social settings. Once you've tried a little in private, go out and see if you can gracefully get through these social cues in public, such as at a restaurant, at a library or store, on public transit, at a ball game.

- Learn the fine art of listening. Remember the tip to study the color of someone's eyes? This helps making eye contact comfortable for both the observer and the person being observed. When you listen to someone, give that person validation if they talk about their emotions. "When he raised his voice at me in front of everyone, I felt so angry, and also ashamed." "Of course, you did! I would, too." Ask the person questions to clarify anything they said.

- Keep your posture straight. If you need physical stimulation to stay focused, you can play with the straw of your drink or subtly tap one finger to your thumb at a time.

- If you're feeling overwhelmed, you can gracefully excuse yourself from the conversation by saying, "Excuse me for a moment. I'm enjoying talking with you, but I have to take care of something really quick." Remember to smile to leave them with a feeling of friendliness and warmth. They might reach out to shake your hand and say "Nice meeting you" or "It was a pleasure". Simply shake their hand, add a smile, and say "Same."

Finally, if you feel like having the support of a community would do you some good, seek out your local autism peer support group. There you can find others who are going through what you are, and who might have additional tips and tricks that have worked for them in social situations.

The Importance of Empathy

One of the biggest fears that haunts many of us in a social environment is the fear that we are being judged. Even if we think that we don't care about this, deep down, being painted unfairly or looked down upon is a very uncomfortable feeling. The key to never make someone feel this way in conversation is to make sure that you have *empathy*. You don't have to state that you empathize with them to let them know it's there—if you feel it, so will they. When you cultivate the ability to see things from someone else's point of view, it makes it easier to bridge the gap from your reality to theirs, and vice versa. Each of us lives and sees life in a unique way. We all may have similarities, but we all have something that's just slightly different about us as well. Having the mindset that being different is not only normal, but interesting and even delightful, will cultivate warmth between you and your conversational partner or group.

Chapter 6 How To Improve Your Listening Skills

Listening is a skill that is critical to the success of the effectiveness of the process of communication. Its importance is heightened in the current context of human interaction where technology has, over time, become a challenge in achieving effective communication. This is particularly true where technology is considered as a distraction. The underlying focus when it comes to improving listening skills is to be patient and to focus on becoming an active listener. Active listening can be defined as listening with full attention. Active listening can also be referred to as a conscious type of listening as it starts with one making a conscious choice to listen actively. With active listening, one overtime gets to see the improvement that is sustainable and predictable. What makes the skill of listening essential is that it is in essence, one giving up a resource they can never take back i.e., the resource of time. Active listening is considered as a psychological tool.

In a world that is highly competitive, the skill of listening can be a tool used to put one or an organization in the leadership position. Leadership that listens is considered as one that is responsive and understanding. This is because when used correctly, listening can improve how accurate an organization or person is in providing value. When an organization adds value, they, in turn, can gain loyalty from their customers, which can mean an increase in business opportunities presented to the organization. Listening well in itself is a tool that can be used to save time by reducing the amount of error likely to occur due to misinterpretation.

The skill of listening is applicable in varied scenarios, including at work and within the context of personal life. The advantages of listening include:

- Having the ability to make one feel heard either as a speaker or an audience. This can be useful in scenarios involving conflict or for effective selling.
- Using the skill to build relationships that are strong.
- Being able to build genuine connections with others.
- Being able to learn new languages.

When one feels heard, one is more likely to express their genuine viewpoint on a myriad of issues. In an environment that requires teamwork, good listening skills are critical in bringing team members into sync. This creates a work environment where solutions and creativity easily flow. Creating a positive work environment via the use of listening skills can mean the difference between retaining good workers and losing them to the competition.

Listening skills can assist individuals in letting go of emotions that are negative in nature. This is exemplified as utilized by counselors during counseling sessions. There are particular skills that one can use in order to listen effectively. These include:

Attention: Part of being a good listener is giving speaker attention by focusing fully on the speaker. This will involve looking at the speaker and watching for cues that are non-verbal in nature that is also referred to as body language. Somebody language cues are placing hands across the chest. The tone of a speaker's voice is also an example of a non-verbal cue. A speaker's tone can give a good listener a glimpse of the emotional state of the speaker. When one does not focus on the speaker, one will miss these cues. Non-verbal cues can give a listener insight into the emotional state of the one speaking. One can try to repeat the words a speaker uses internally in one's head as a means of keeping the focus on a speaker. The act of such repetition allows one to reinforce the message that the speaker is trying to get across.

When giving speaker attention, be sure to do so with balance, so that the speaker does not interpret the attention as staring or intimidation. Also, one should try to individualize the attention specific to the emotions of the speaker. To be a listener who gets the whole picture of the message being transmitted, one must process both the verbal and non-verbal in tandem. Depending on where communication is taking place, the listener might have to mentally get rid of any sort of distractions e.g., background activity. Distractions can be internal or external. Internal ones include one's thought pattern moving away from what a speaker is saying.

It is also important to individualize the type of attention to give as what may be considered as attention in one set e.g., eye contact may be considered rude in another culture. Giving cues to show one is attentive is more important than the type of cue.

Avoid deflection: Deflection can be defined as pushing back or away from. In the context of developing effective listening skills, it is exemplified when a listener makes the decision to move the topic of conversation from the one the speaker is currently on, to one that is of interest to them. This may be due to the listener being uncomfortable or even bored with the topic at hand. It would be more subtle to use close-ended questions to shorten the message of the speaker than to change the topic outrightly. The skill to be developed here is to subtly encourage the speaker to move away from the topic at hand without taking over the process of doing so.

From the speaker's point of view, a listener who chooses to deflect comes off as one who has no respect for them or even one who is selfish.

Avoid outsmarting: To become a good listener, one must refrain from taking the focus from the speaker to themselves. One of the ways one does this is by choosing to share a scenario where one faced the same situation as the one that the speaker is trying to share. This portrays the listener as one who is boastful and selfish.

Avoid setting judgments: This involves one holding back from being critical of the one they are listening to. This way, one gives themselves a chance to see a situation from the viewpoint of the speaker. In some scenarios, using this tool to improve listening may end up allowing an unexpected connection to occur between the most unlikely of people, even as they take note of the similarities between them. One should avoid voicing criticisms while listening as the speaker may decide to stop communicating. Generally, when one entertains critical thoughts as they are listening, the same shows up via non-verbal cues e.g., through frowning. The non-verbal negative cues can cause the speaker to become defensive, leading to ineffective communication.

Not judging can also help one not to come up with preconceived conclusions that may change the perception of what the message was intended to be. Passing judgments can also be in the form of mentally correcting one's accent or spelling. Doing so distracts one from forming the habit of effective listening.

Big picture: When listening to a speaker, one should aim to focus on the overall message as opposed to the details, as the latter may lead to unnecessary distractions that lead one to miss out on what was the focus of the message that the speaker wanted the listener to get. In a one-on-one setting, allowing distractions may force the one listening to ask a speaker to repeat themselves. This may cause the speaker to feel frustrated and may portray the listener as one who is disinterested in the message being passed. Unnecessary repetitions due to the lack of focus on the side of the listener are also time-wasting.

When one focuses on the big picture, they may also be less critical, therefore becoming more effective at listening. When one is less critical, one focuses on the content shared in communication as opposed to mistakes perceived as having occurred.

Context: To be an effective listener, one must always put into view the context within which a message is being transmitted. The same message can have varied meanings in different contexts.

Culture: Effective listeners are culturally aware. One being culturally aware allows for one to use tools for effective listening within a cultural context productively. Being unaware of culture may inhibit effective communication. This is because what one culture considers appropriate, another may consider insulting.

Emotions: Connecting with the emotions that a speaker displays or is feeling makes one a great listener. Doing so can allow the listener to be empathetic to the speaker. In some cases, it can lead to the building of a successful relationship between the speaker and the listener. This relationship can then be leveraged for other situations. The speaker will be able to tell when a listener connects to them emotionally, via the mirroring of emotions that will take place via non-verbal cues on the part of the listener. For one to identify with the emotions of a speaker, one has to have their full attention on the speaker, which in turn makes one a better listener as they are actively listening.

One way a good listener connects with a speaker is by amplifying the emotions that the speaker displays.

Facing: Depending on the cultural context, it is advisable to face one in whom one is in communication with. This implies interest, confidence, and in some scenarios, respect. It also gives the speaker the indication or go-ahead to start or continue communicating. Looking away from the speaker may signify the opposite. When facing one speaking, be sure to get rid of distractions. What one should remember when using the tool of facing to become an effective listener is that they are to do this without portraying a confrontational posture.

Feedback: To be a good listener, one must learn the art of giving feedback. Feedback can be given either verbally or non-verbally. Generally, the non-verbal aspect makes up the bigger composition of communication. I am giving feedback signals to the speaker that one is attentive and interested in the message being transmitted. Giving feedback also helps a listener stay attentive. In the context of feedback, the listener should aim to mirror the feelings of the one they are listening to. Feedback can be in the form of paraphrasing, which helps in ensuring the listener and the one speaking are on the same page. Paraphrasing is also a way through which the listener demonstrates to the speaker how well they can listen.

Giving feedback can also help to avoid misunderstandings, which if not dealt with, would lead to ineffective communication. Feedback can also be a way through which a listener can communicate to a speaker that they have understood the message transmitted. One should be aware though, that the feedback given should portray that one is listening yet not necessarily that they are in agreement with the message being transmitted. The feedback should focus on acknowledgment as opposed to the agreement unless the listener actually agrees with the message being communicated. When giving non-verbal feedback, the listener should use one that is comfortable to them, yet take into account the cultural context of where the communication is occurring. This is to ensure that they don't look or feel awkward or portray a message to the speaker that is varied from their intended communication.

Giving feedback may also reduce on time wastage, as the one speaking may not feel the need to repeat their message, as a way of being sure that the one listening has understood the message that the speaker had intended to communicate. When giving feedback verbally, a good listener should not repeat word for word what the speaker says, but instead, rephrase the message communicated. The focus here is to give feedback on the listener's own words. It is also important for a good listener to give feedback at the appropriate time. The appropriate time is dependent on the context within which the communication is occurring. One can sometimes tell that it is an appropriate time to share feedback by studying the cues given by the speaker. Some cues here can include the speaker pausing or looking at the listener for evidence that they are being heard.

Another point to consider when giving feedback is that the response should fully be about the speaker. A good listener will not include themselves in the feedback by e.g., using words that would be inclusive of them like the word we. When using rephrasing for feedback, it is best for the ownership of the rephrase to be the listener. The rule of thumb in regards to feedback, though the context should be considered, is that it should be shorter than the message received from the speaker.

To avoid being critical in the context of feedback, one should aim not to let their own value systems and biases block their ability to listen actively.

Goal: To be effective at listening, one should come up with a practical goal for the same. A goal in listening effectively can be that one will only speak a quarter of the time and listen to the rest of the time that the communication process is taking place. The use of this tool, though, it must be applied in the context of how and where the communication process occurs. The overall goal generally would be to speak less and listen more.

Growth: A way of becoming a good listener is to consider listening as an opportunity for growth. Humans have had different experiences in life, can be a source of learning if only one truly listens. Having a growth viewpoint in the context of listening will be portrayed even in your non-verbal or body language positively. The growth viewpoint may also give one information on how to deal with issues in a different manner. Listening can be an aid in the journey of personal growth or self-development.

Hear: To be an effective listener, one should always put themselves in a position to actually hear what the speaker is communicating. This may mean adjusting the volume or requesting that the speaker increase how loud they are speaking. It may also mean the listener needs to get rid of distractions or even draw closer in proximity to where the speaker is. If at all the listening part is being affected by something that needs medical attention, one should aim to seek for help if possible, in order to become effective at listening.

Interrupt minimally: Interrupting an individual as they speak may lead to them getting frustrated. They end up with the feeling of not being understood nor heard and even disrespected. These feelings can lead to obstacles against effective communication occurring. Depending on the context, the speaker may decide to stop communicating. The speaker may interpret the interruption as a show of rudeness, which may end up destroying a relationship. Also, an interruption can be in the form of trying to predict verbally what the other party is trying to say. This has a presumption that the listener can read in advance the thoughts and feelings of the speaker.

Doing so can lead to a myriad of misunderstandings. It may also project to the one speaking that the listener is impatient. Interruptions give a feeling of a contest where two parties are competing for who should be heard. This does not augur well with the goal of building relationships through active listening. To avoid being a source of interruption to one speaking one can choose to:

- *Practice having one's mouth stay shut during listening. When an individual chooses to focus on keeping their mouth closed, they can end up becoming better at listening.*

- *Take notes of what one considers to be important points raised by the speaker. Also, one can put down points that one considers of importance that come to mind as they listen to the one speaking. The other party may consider it a sign of respect when someone puts down what they are saying as it means that it is important to the listener. It should* be noted though, that some speakers interpret this action as evidence of the listener being distracted, and may, therefore, discourage it.

• Change where one's attention is at. This is about placing attention on the aspect of listening as opposed to the one of speaking or responding as the case might be. One can also choose to come up with a goal to talk less than they speak at any given time.

Chapter 7 How to Attract and Keep Great Friends

Have you ever wondered why some people attract and make friends easily? Maybe you thought there is something that they are doing differently that if you could put your fingers on would help you meet loving, close, fulfilling friends. The secret to making friendship is how people think. Those who get many friends are always positive thinkers who focus on things that make them happy and feel better about themselves. This allows them to have a welcoming and open vibration that makes others want to stick around them. In this chapter, we discuss how we can attract and keep great friends

How To Attract True Friends?

The difference between your current position and your future is greatly influenced by the people you hang around. Friends are capable of influencing, changing, and convincing us. Because of this, attracting friends who have a positive influence in our lives is very important, and requires few skills that should not be overlooked. By implementing the tips below, you will be able to attract great friends.

1. Always be yourself

Good friends are those who love you for who you are and accept you the way you are. They never mind about your flaws, and they will never try to change you into someone else. They say, "birds of the same feathers flock together" is a reflection of true and real friendship. When you reveal your true personality, you will only attract those who are fascinated with such character and personality.

Never be shy to express your fantasies and exploring your hobbies. When you are around people, talk about the things that you love, and this way, you will only attract those who have the same interest.

2. Don't try too hard to fit in

Being a kind person is humane. However, being too kind can be detrimental to your peace of mind and your well-being. If you make it a habit of being too kind, and always in the habit of pleasing everybody, your life span will be too short. Most "friends" may turn sour when they realize you do not answer yes to all their requests. The right friends are those who value you regardless of any situation and can never be bought by your good deeds. Great friends are always comfortable airing their opinions with you without compromise and are only attracted to those who are bold enough to act or speak their minds.

3. Set your standards and stick to them

Principles and standards prevent unwanted people from our lives. Principles are the things we hold to be true to follow. They guide and govern our lives along different paths. It is important to distinguish what views are right or positive from those that are obscene or wrong. With such standards, you will be able to restrict your friendship to only those who have particular behaviors that go with your values and beliefs.

4. Always develop yourself

In order to attract the right friends, you must be good yourself. Friendship is never about what you gain or pursue from the other person, but rather it is about the contributions you make to their wellbeing and prosperity. You can never contribute to someone's life positively if you have never invested in yourself first. This means that you must be the best version of yourself to grow.

Ways To Keep Great Friends

Just like any other relationship, every friendship requires importance, care, tie, and dedication. It is important that you maintain your friendship for it to last longer. Below I have highlighted the seven ways through which you can attract friends and keep them for life.

Have the three-word question at your fingertips

An important question that we need to ask our friends is, 'How are you?' But few of us care to really listen to the response. This question shows that one truly cares for the other person, and wish to know how their lives are faring. Everyone has become conditioned to this greeting that the words have actually lost the meaning. So, you could add follow-up questions such as "what have you been up to?" "How are your children?" or "how is your partner" to get more specific details.

Consider friendship as an investment

Friendship is just as important as healthy life like fitness and diet is, and so should be treated in a similar manner. Just like fitness goals would fade away if taken for granted, friendships fade away if you do not nurture them. Consider your friendships as an investment for your future. With social media availability, you are able to check on your friends and even meet new ones. You should also create enough time for physical connection; if not in person, you may interact through FaceTime, Skype, or similar tools.

Always ask questions and listen to the answers

One of the best ways to connect with people is through asking questions and listening to the answers given carefully. Most people ask questions but fail to listen to the answers, and instead impatiently wait for their turn to speak. Without proper listening, you are not capable of building a conversation, which would jeopardize your chances of making a genuine connection. It is important that you listen properly, pick up something from their talk, and develop even further conversation. As you listen, consider using nonverbal cues such as nodding and making listening sounds like 'go on,' 'really,' 'hmm', and 'tell me more."

Share your story

Although listening is the best way to have a genuine connection with other people, you should be willing to share things about yourself too. A great friendship is built on the commonalities and similarities existing between people; so, you should be able to share yours. However, ensure that you are only sharing the necessary details and that the dialogue remains equally shared.

Provide genuine compliments

Offer compliments that reveal your genuineness. Do not just say, "you look good," say, "I really like your skirt and makeup." Unless you are connecting with a stoker, you need to ensure that your compliments focus on authentic similarities so that you appear genuine. Potential friends can easily be repelled by fake compliments.

Be authentic

If you want to make friends, you need to look for things that draw attention to your commonalities. When conversing and you find yourself using statements like, "I get it," "I understand what you mean," or "I thought so too," it is obvious that your experiences are on the same wavelength. Be enthusiastic and open, behave in a friendly manner, smile, and act like you really enjoy life.

Chapter 8 Looking at Things From A New Angle

Whether it is conflict or decision-making, understanding how things appear at a different angle is beneficial. It helps to be interactive and inclusive. Differences may exist between people and partners in a social, family, or working relationship. When this occurs, it is necessary to do less political strategizing and more thinking of different angles for solutions. Being able to look at things from a new angle requires three skills: perspective-taking, perspective-seeking, and perspective-coordinating.

1) Perspective-taking

Perspective-taking is a critical component of communication. Depending on where we stand, the way we perceive facts and their meaning can be very different. The perspective we adopt influences what we consider obvious or obscure, central or peripheral, and present or absent. Just like the way we perceive the physical world; perspective influences the human experience in the social world. If we can see things in a different angle, from the perspective of another person, we can have responses that are more constructive rather than several strong disagreements. At the least, we can be careful in what we do or say in challenging times to avoid escalating negative outcomes.

Mistaking perspective-taking

When we are trying to look at things from a different angle, we should avoid two pitfalls: overconfidence and uncritically considering another person's view as valid. More often, we get overconfident that we are succeeding in viewing things from a different perspective. Remember a time your friend was displeased with the birthday gift you bought her or doubly upset for not understanding her troubles. The fact is that you may have tried to take their perspective but ended up with a mistaken one.

Studies have revealed that people are often inaccurate when they infer the thoughts and feelings of another person by observing the behaviors and facial expressions of that person. More important, people become overconfident that they finally managed to get a different perspective right.

Another common pitfall is the idea that most people treat another person's perspective as valid, thereby using it to solve a problem. When our perspectives are based on wrong assumptions, the effect is missing the real issues or misleading conclusion. An example is a leader making judgments on an incident with the assumption that he/she had access to the critical information for decision-making. However, if the assumption is wrong and not questioned, then the judgment could end up solving an integrity issue when the real one could be information quality.

2) Perspective-seeking

To successfully view things from a new angle, you also need to have the skill of perspective-seeking. Once one is able to listen to other people's perspective, they should be able to judge whether it is right or wrong. This skill involves understanding another person's point of view on a particular point or circumstance. It is about being curious to hear and learn more about other perspectives.

The greatest trap on this skill is reaching out to people with a similar point of view that you have in order to validate a hard decision you plan to make. It is important to listen to people who may have a different opinion from yours and discover new things as well as potential blind spots.

3) Perspective-coordinating

Once you can take different perspectives and seek them out, you need the perspective-coordinating skill in order to utilize the information you received. Perspective-coordinating entails observing what lessons are available from the other perspectives. This skill helps us to understand other people we speak to and the impact of our final decisions on them. Also, perspective-coordinating enables one to understand the contributions of different viewpoints in every situation and how they help in decision-making.

How to Radically Look at Things From a New Angle

Perspective-taking not only brings empathy in our social relationships, but it also brings in compassion and mindfulness of the people we connect with. Below are the ways through which you can successfully view things in a new angle by considering other people's views.

Think of others

When we are in the presence of other people, we naturally begin to think about what they are thinking. We observe their behaviors, such as where they are looking, what they are doing, and their body language. This observation helps us to determine whether we can be comfortable around them or have further association with them. If you think about other people and feel comfortable around them, we begin to think of how to connect with them. The information you get by observing others will prompt you to speak up in a conversation and get to learn their perspective.

Regulate your emotions and empathy

Taking perspective depends on our ability to share emotions as well as the capacity to regulate our emotions. In order to be effective with other people, we must understand the things that trigger us so that we can refocus ourselves in time on what is happening to others. In regard to empathy, we should try to understand what other people would do in a particular situation rather than what we would do.

With stronger empathic accuracy and emotional regulation skills, you can be successful in considering different perspectives. The skills can help you to predict expectations, intentions, and attitudes of others, which may be different from your own.

Reading others correctly

Our perspective-taking guides are the emotions, which help us to read and learn people. Our eye and brains help us to track the behaviors of others and determine what they are feeling or thinking, then determining their intentions and motives. By being sensitive to other people, you will be able to sense their possible emotional changes, which can help in gauging how to successfully show up in the interaction.

4. Interpret words

Most people do not speak directly, which often requires that we infer the mean of what they are trying to say. However, this always creates a lot of room for misinterpreting the message, particularly those sent via email or text. By accurately interpreting what the other person is saying, you will be able to make the right decision on what to say and avoid conflict.

5. Respect the existing differences

To take the perspectives of other people, we need to have the maturity to respect the personal beliefs of others and respect their knowledge. If we disrespect others, they will separate themselves from us and avoid sharing their constructive ideas with us. It is important to be highly attuned that people hold different beliefs and world views, and as such, remain open-minded and respectful as we interact with them.

6. Be interactive

We must interact with people in order to develop empathy and learn from their ideas. Interactions are made possible by asking questions and listening to find out the concerns and experiences of other people. When individuals engage in naturalistic connections, they can tell each other what they truly think rather than what the other person wants to hear. As a result, this opens up doors to learning new perspectives.

Quality interactions build social cohesion, promote mutual trust, and reciprocity norms. Over time, these traits motivate people to see things from others' perspectives, promote collaboration, and facilitate conflict resolution.

7. Strike a balance between subjectivity and objectivity

To empathize with the perspective of another person, you need to actively adopt that perspective with subjectivity and emotions. But note that empathy should be accompanied by certain level of detachment to maintain objectivity for effect perspective evaluation. Detachment refers to the ability of an individual to step back from an idea in order to see the bigger picture. This way, we can learn other people's perspective and apply them adequately.

Chapter 9 Broaden Your Horizons

Broadening your horizons always means experiencing or learning something you have never known before, and opening yourself up for new ideas. There are several ways to expand our horizons, but the most common metaphor used is usually through traveling. Although traveling is a big part of life accompanied by a lot of experiences, the metaphor means so much more. Expanding horizons require courage. You must leave your comfort zone to learn or try something new, which may be difficult in a society where people are okay with following the status quo. In this chapter, you are going to learn about the amazing ways to broaden your horizons and the people you should surround yourself with to expand the horizons.

Amazing Ways to Broaden Your Horizons

Stop limiting yourself. Often, we get stuck from exploring because we believe in false barriers. Whether you believe something because someone told you it's the "truth" or from your own experience, notions that limit you can prevent you from living a complete, fulfilling life. Self-limiting factors are those things we can never challenge; we just consider them truthful even if they are not. For example, if you believe that you cannot possibly swim, then you may probably never swim. In this case, you limit your ability with the belief that you are unable to.

Keep constantly pushing yourself. Broadening one's horizon is never an easy task. We do things in a particular manner when they are predictable, and the outcomes are not scary. If you wish to broaden your horizons, you must put in extra efforts, work harder, and be able to invest more time and go an extra mile. If you do this, the rewards will be much better than a simple part on the back for a job done well.

Move away from your comfort zone. Most of the time, we don't do things in life because they are not "comfortable." This means that they make us uneasy and out of control. If you want to broaden your horizons, you must be willing to keep going even without feeling safe and not knowing how the process will end. This does not, however, mean that you put yourself in the harm's way, but it means putting yourself in the awkward, weird, and persevering position. Since everyone can adapt to feeling uncomfortable, you should not be scared of the risks.

Be quiet and listen. We are always busy telling others about ourselves or how things are going that we forget to stop and listen. In order to broaden your horizons, you need to listen to others and challenger your own beliefs. If you spend all your time trying to convince people that you are always right, you will never stop to consider their own ideas and perspectives. Broadening horizons require that you keep quiet and let someone else talk. You may ask questions later to get more information that would help in expanding your horizons.

Ask yourself why. The older you get, the more you will realize that the things you thought you knew might actually not be the case. Personally, I have gone through being a Republican to a Democrat and back again many times. If you believe in a particular political system, you might have asked yourself several times why you accept that without having any reason behind it. The moment you stop asking yourself questions, you will have stopped growing. To broaden your horizons, you have to stop believing everything as facts and ask questions about them.

Do the opposite. Doing the exact opposite of the things you always do is another way of expanding your horizons. When you see two people having an exchange, consider the devil's advocate position and go with it. When you normally go left, take a right this time. If you always swim on weekends, consider going to a dancing lesson or hiking. The change with impact all your life experiences and further enhance your thoughts.

Develop empathy. If you want to broaden your horizons, it is important to be in someone else's shoes. Look around and see what you have that others do not have. Often, we make a lot of effort to convince people that we deserve what we have, that we forget to see that others are deserving as well. This limits the way we carry out ourselves and the life we live.

The 5 People You Need in Life to Broaden your Horizons

If you choose to only surround yourself with people who have the same background as you, same age group, and same circumstance, you will be leading a boring, homogenous life without new things or ideas to explore. Your perspectives will be limited to the group of people you associate with. Variety is the spice of life and having versatile people can expose you to different lifestyles that you may not have considered before. Thus, if you need to broaden your horizons, consider associating yourself with the following people:

The wise guru: Many young people immerse themselves in the belief that they cannot have friends with people who are older than them. They believe that older people cannot relate to anything they are going through. But this is not the case; they were your once, too! It is important to have wise friends who are older than you are to share their perspectives, life experiences, and wisdom. Always smile with your elderly neighbors, take some cookies to your grandparents, and have regular kickback sessions with some of your elderly church members. These people can impact your life by sharing their stories and wisdom.

The "Phoebe": These are people with free spirits always willing to go an extra mile in pushing you to further your limits. They are friends that convince you to take a last-minute trip to another country, and who will remind you to never take life too seriously. It is in their nature to seek adventure, live in the moment, and view life through rose-colored glasses. Such people will make you enjoy life as they challenge you to engage in challenging tasks.

The over-achiever: These are the types of friends who made it to the varsity and graduated with honors. They work very hard and earn a lot of money, while still getting enough time to volunteer to charity organizations on the weekend. They are so disciplined and incredibly collected together. Instead of being jealous of them, it is important to embrace such people as they will encourage you to become a champion in life. Learn their habits and behaviors, and ask them to teach you the ways to success.

The mentee: Mentoring a younger person will give you the happiness and joy you need to grow in life. Mentoring someone gives you the chance to be a much-needed positive influence on someone as well as remind you how to strive towards success. Become a mentor at your former school, volunteer at a community home, or simply help your cousin or daughter with homework. Mentees help you to expand your horizon to get even more influential.

The person in the mirror: Nothing can broaden your perspective than actually getting to know yourself. While growing, we tend to care about making new friends and wondering about what the world thinks of us. However, we always end up neglecting ourselves in the process. You cannot fulfill your potential if you fail to discover yourself. Spend time alone, treat yourself solo to a vacation, journal, or treat yourself by going for a hangout at the coffee shop. These gestures not only expand your mind but also lift your spirits for future adventures.

Chapter 10 Social/Communication Skills At Job Interviews

You have come too far to mess things up. You have done a lot of research, spent your time to gather all that you need for the interview, and even groomed yourself for the occasion. It would be a pity to lose it all for mistakes you did on the actual interview. Remember the objective of your interview is to land a job offer. To realize this objective, you will, by all means, have to prove that you are the best there is. If you are waiting to do big things to blow away your hiring managers, it is time to wake up and smell the coffee. It is the little things that matter and that will possibly work for you or against you.

What to do during the interview

Be on time

You cannot afford to be late to an interview. Arriving early acts as proof that you are time conscious. Before the interview though, you should call to inform the hiring managers what time they should expect you.

But while arriving early to an interview is an added plus, you should not by any means be there thirty minutes to the start of the interview. As a matter of fact, it is recommended that you be at the interview location at most 15 minutes before the start of the interviews. Getting to your destination too early could work against you. Rather than calming down to compose yourself, you will start to freak out after your brain starts to work overtime thinking of all scary and imaginary scenarios.

If for some reason beyond your control you will be arriving late, be sure to call and inform your contact. This shows responsibility and maturity qualities that will earn you points.

Say Hi to the receptionist

It is common courtesy to greet people you meet. You do not have to start up a conversation, as a matter of fact; it is not recommended that you do. If you can, also get his/her name if it is not on a tag somewhere. This is very important since some hiring managers seek to see just how keen you are and aware of your environment or even friendliness by asking you the name of the receptionist or even the guard at the door.

Which might seem harsh but valid? Hiring managers do not want to hire robots or persons who say they are friendly and do not care enough to know the name of the receptionist or even the guard.

Have the right body language

Your body language will communicate just as much as the information you offer to your hiring managers. You do not want to be in a situation that you say you are confident but your body language reeks of lacking in confidence. Try as much as you can to have your body language convey the same message as your words. If you say you are confident, do maintain an upright posture, maintain eye contact and have a convincing tone.

If slouching, fidgeting and looking down are bad habits that you possess, you can get rid of them by practicing in front of a mirror. Pull up a chair and observe your body language.

Also, avoid flattering behaviors like biting your lower lip or winking. You might be unaware that you wink at people or it is just something you picked up over the years, regardless, you might have to actively subdue them.

Have the right tone of voice

Like your body language, your tone will also speak a thousand words. You could repeat that you know how to do your job a thousand times but if you do not sound like you can, your words are worth nothing. Have a tone that will inspire confidence in your hiring manager.

So, how does one sound more confident during a job interview?

Take your time to think over the question, gather your thoughts before you answer. The recommended time to take for this is five seconds. Now it might seem like such a long time and awkwardness might set in but the interviewer sees it as you giving your answer some consideration.

Always have an interested tone though factual and straight forward. You should keep away from raising your pitch towards the end of your statements as this will turn them into questions making you seem uncertain of what you are saying. You should however vary your tone depending on the question and what it relates to. Do not overdo it though.

Do not apologize for being nervous. Doing this will actually put more scrutiny on just how worried you are about your performance.

Use a firm handshake

There are individuals who are sucker for firm handshakes. There are those who can tell who you are from the way you shake their hand. Just ensure you do not hurt your hiring manager while you are at it.

Dress appropriately

If you are dressed too casually or too formal, things will be very uncomfortable for you. It is important to know the dress code of the company you are interviewing at beforehand for the sake of this planning.

Sit only when you are asked to

When you walk into the room, only take a seat when they ask you to and not before. It is a sign of politeness. It is the same thing as when someone is at your door. They should wait until you invite them in (especially if you are not as close).

Have your loose items on the floor right next to you

You should never place your items on the interviewer desk unless they say that it is okay that you do so. Have all these items placed comfortably on your lap or on a coffee table right in front of you. As for your briefcase, have it right at your feet or on your side.

Have your mobile turned off

You do not want to have disruptions during the interview. Setting your phone to vibrate just won't cut it.

Thank your interviewer

The fact that they choose you out of the hundreds and thousands of applicants is worth saying thank you,

What not to do during an interview

Do not assume the interview is done until you are out of the door

From the moment you walk in the office the interview is on. Everything from your behavior, use of words to attitude is under scrutiny. As such, you should be overly careful of what you say. After all, everything you say and do will be held and used against you. Be at the very top of our game until you walk out that door, or better yet, out of the company building. You never know who you will bump into on your way out so be respectful to everyone.

Do not be too relaxed

Sure, the interview is a platform for you to gauge is you will love the job and you are encouraged to be relaxed. You should however not treat your hiring manager like your long-lost friend (even if he/she is). You should be friendly, but remember you are seeking to be impressive. Being too relaxed may have you slipping up and saying the wrong things altogether.

Never badmouth your old job

Maybe your former boss was the devil incarnate and is probably the reason why you left your past job. But be it as it may, you should not point it out to your hiring manager. As far as your hiring company is concerned, you should get along with everyone you are given to work with no matter how difficult they are. So rather than badmouth your previous boss or company, speak of the achievements you made as a team. Doing this will also keep you from coming across as self-centered.

Do not freak out if you do not know the answer

Some hiring managers are known for putting their interviewees on the spot. And since you never know what kind of hiring manager you will get, you should always be prepared. Never freak out when you are presented with a question that you do not know the answer to. Freaking out will make you lose all sense of rationality making things even worse. So how should you hand yourself in such a situation?

First, and most important, you should calm down. Freaking out will rise your heart beat rate, rise your temperature and cloud your judgments. Be sure to take deep breaths and convince yourself that all is well. After all, it is okay not to know the answer to a question.

Second, even when you do not know the answer to the question provided, never say that you do not know the answer without giving it a try. Also, as you try to give your answer, do not make things up. Hiring managers are not stupid and will be sure to see right through the crap.

You also have the option of asking follow up questions to ensure you understand the question right. Ask for clarification and more details that will help you provide a better answer.

But even after the clarification, if the question still proves difficult to answer, be sure to iterate what you do know rather than what you do not know. Also, you should spell out the steps that you could take to get to the answer of the question presented. This way, even while you may not have the answer at the moment, you assure the hiring managers that you have the ability to get to the answer if afforded more time.

Never lie

You should, by all means, be straight forward with your hiring manager. It is as they say, the truth always has a way of coming out. When lying, you may not be able to hold a sincere flowing conversation with the hiring manager and this might be a major turn off. Truth be told, honesty is the best policy. Even when you land that job position you will have started on the wrong foot and it is only a matter of time before your lies catch up with you.

Avoid talking about your problems

Sure, you need the job do get several things in your life going. You need to pay off that student loan, you need to put food on the table for your family, you need to get your child through college and a host of other financial responsibilities that you have. But think about it are you the only one with these responsibilities? No. In an interview, you should not go to personal as to why you need the nob. Do not try to land the job by preying on the pity of the hiring managers. Rather, show them how strong and confident you are and just why they cannot do without you. Doing this, you will land the job and comfortably cater to your 101 problems.

Cursing

You probably are used to foul language. But as you probably already know, this is unacceptable in a job interview. It shows a lack of respect and regard for everyone around you.

Never say that you do not have the experience

The fact that the company called you in for an interview is evidence enough that they consider you to be qualified enough for the job position. It is up to you to give them that final nudge or push they need to give you an offer.

If you are a recent graduate, you probably are feeling not up to the task of the position available. Going through the list of responsibilities made everything worse. All those tasks and duties looked all so daunting. Before you think to yourself how inexperienced you are, know one thing, many people learn on the job and you are just what they need. Do not focus on your weaknesses but rather keep your focus on your strengths.

How to Answer Questions you may be asked in an interview

How great it would be to have all the questions you will be asked in an interview? Knowing every question and being prepared for it. Well, you can have a preview of some questions you should expect and just how you should approach their answers. But while this is here to help you, you should not give he answers word forward. Use these questions and answers as a guide to get to know how to recreate your own curate, sincere responses.

Can you tell me about yourself?

From face value, this question is probably one here is. But one that many people fail for lack of preparation. Here is how you go about answering this question. It might be tempting, but you should not go into personal history details. You should however make your answer more of a pitch. A pitch that is compelling and concise showing just how you are the perfect fit for the job position. You could start specifying your experiences and accomplishments in brief and target them to just how you the company can benefit from having you.

What information do you know about the company?

Anyone can memorize the company about us page and spit it out like spoken word or a poem. So, when the hiring managers ask about it, they are not looking to know whether you know the mission statement word forward or the company core values, they just want to know whether you care about it and if they are in line with what you believe in.

So rather than spit it out word for word, start by showing you understands the company goals. You can throw in a few keywords from the company site after which you can make a follow up with why you are drawn to the mission statement and probably why you believe in the approach they are taking as a business.

Why do you want this job?

Companies want people who are passionate about what they do and consequently the job position that they have open. You should as such have one of the best answers for this particular question. To provide the best answer for this, you should identify some of the reasons you think you are the perfect fit for the job position you have applied to. If it is customer service, probably you are great with people and providing satisfactory answers to them is easy and you love helping out people. Also, explain just why you love the company.

Why should we hire you?

These questions seem intimidating and for the most part rude and arrogant. But when you look at it in depth, it actually is not. Yes, it is forward and all, but you should count it as a benefit and count yourself lucky. It is a one of a kind opportunity served to you hot on a silver platter; an opportunity to sell yourself. As you are answering this question, pay attention to three main point, the fact that you can not only get the job done but you can also deliver the best possible results and that you fit in just fine with any group regardless of the diversity.

What do you consider your weakness?

The employer is trying to flash out any red flags and gauge your honesty and self-awareness. As such, even while you are advised to be honest in an interview, you cannot say that you cannot meet deadlines even when my life is on the line. You also cannot say that you are perfect. Weaseling out of the question is not an option that you have.

Here is how you go about this question. Strive a perfect balance with the things that you are struggling with and the things that you know you should work on improving. For instance, you may not be the best public speaker, but you have been volunteering to speak in meetings to get comfortable with the whole scenario.

Special interview scenarios

Not all interviews will be conducted behind closed doors at the office. There are those that are conducted over the phone, those that are over lunch or breakfast and others that are group interviews. While the basics of acing an interview remain, there are some variations.

Phone interviews

In most interviewing process, this is never a final interview. It acts as a preliminary and to get a first impression of whether or not you should be hired. It is as such important that you bring your A game.

Aside from being prepared, practicing beforehand and knowing everything there is to know about the company, you should;

Ensure you have a quiet environment

Turn off the radio and television. Get yourself a quiet spot if you have family and friends around. You might let you family and friends know that you will be having an interview at a particular time so that they provide you with the space you need.

Remain calm

Before answering the phone, take deep breaths and smile. The interviewer will not see your smile but this will have a great effect on the tone of voice that you have during the interview. It will be happy confident. If you a tricky question is asked, take your time to think about it. Be sure not to wait too long though.

Be professional

You know when the interview will be conducted right? You also know the number they will use to call. As such, while picking up the call you should ensure that you are as professional as you can be. Good morning/evening, Kevin Fikes speaking will do the trick.

Meal interviews

As for meal interviews, there are more of things you should not do

Do not start selling yourself immediately. Let the hiring manager lead the conversation. Your job is to ensure that you have a sincere and flowing conversation. The selling yourself part might come at the end of the meal.

When ordering your food, do not be overly picky. Pick from the menu being sure to stay away from foods you are allergic to, garlic and onions. Ensure that you have lots of water and have food that you can take with great ease and that is not messy.

Do not talk too much. Interviewers love to make use of what people call the pregnant pause. It is fascinating what stupid and shocking things say in this time. When you are done answering a question, remain quiet.

Do not order the most expensive food in the restaurant. Order what you normally would be sure to keep the costs reasonable. Rather than have dessert, skip to the tea or coffee if they interviewer orders it first. This will show that you are fiscally responsible and that you are not the type to take advantage of the situation.

Group meetings

When you are feeling all prepared and walk right into an office only to find ten more candidates waiting, what should you do?

First, have your poker face on. You might be surprised and your mind might be working overtime but you should not let others see. It. If anything, be confident, or at least fake it with your body language and your look.

Do not be like the rest. Many who get into job interviews tend to go mute and ignore each other. Many even pull out their phones and start playing games or chatting. You should however avoid this, strike a conversation with someone even when the employer is not in the room. Your interaction will show that you do not shy away from a chance to network.

Involve the others rather than treat them as the competition that they are. If you have a chance to talk and elaborate something, you can bring in the others and even mention them by name. This will identify you as the group leader and better placed to land the job.

Also, be sure to add to the points already made by your colleagues. Give it more oomph as you add more thoughts on it.

But above all, you should be yourself. Do not go overboard. Do not try to force situations as this will make you come across as aggressive. While you want to outdo the others, you should not speak over others or discredit their opinions.

Chapter 11 Understand People Emotions

The definition of motivation involves three concepts: Willingness, effort and goals. Willingness is when a person is agreeable towards engaging in a goal-motivated behavior. Effort is the amount of work a person invests towards a goal. Goal is the end, or the result, of someone's striving. Understanding these components and their role in motivation is essential towards understanding how our goals in life become aligned based on our feelings and emotions. Understand that there is one common characteristic though—that all behavior is motivated by something.

Let's start by quickly going through the different theories of motivation and seeing where feelings and emotions come into play.

Instinct Theories of Motivation

These theories have a common denominator: That all people engage in goal-directed behavior because they are programmed with evolution. These theories were widely accepted until the 1920s before other motivational theories were proposed.

A notable proponent of instinct theories was William James. He came up with a list of human instincts that included play, attachment, anger, fear, modesty, love and shyness. At this point, note that anger and fear are emotions while love is a feeling.

Incentive Theory of Motivation

Rewards are at play under this theory as it proposes that people's behavior is motivated by incentives.

Drive Theory of Motivation

More on the biological aspect, this theory proposes that people get their motivations from unsatisfied needs. This can be illustrated by a behavior that seeks to get water because of thirst. However, a certain degree of criticality is involved in this theory. Some people can still eat even when they are not really hungry.

Arousal Theory of Motivation

This theory says that we strive to maintain a subjective level of arousal. This subjective level can be referred to as a sense of equilibrium. When we perceive an imbalance in our arousal levels, we seek to make it optimal. Hence, if we have a high level of arousal, we seek to do activities that will lower it and when our arousal level is low, we tend to engage in behavior that brings it up.

Humanistic Theory of Motivation

Directly related to Abraham Maslow's Hierarchy of Needs, the humanistic theory of motivation states that people have cognitive reasons in performing their actions. This explains why we move from one specific goal to another such that we fulfill our biological needs first before moving on to greater goals like self-actualization.

Bringing it All Together

In our lives, we are made to choose over two or more goals. Our choice, plus the order in which we approach things to achieve the goal are summed up based on our needs and what we want. This concept falls under prioritization. When we prioritize, or make our choices, there is a perceived conflict that happens within us. This is accurately captured under the concept of conflict. This concept proposes one idea that determines our emotions and feelings: That we approach an attractive goal (Approach Process) and that we stay away from an undesirable goal (Avoidance Process). But where do emotions and feelings come in?

The Approach Process

When we approach a goal, we generally perceive it as something beneficial or beautiful. Anything that helps us improve or live better is something considered "approachable." However, the timeline between our initial goal-directed behavior and the goal itself is marred by challenges. Hence, we change our behavior and this change can lead to two results:

If we do poorly, we experience sadness and depression.

If we do well, we experience eagerness and elation.

If we do it just right, we are in a neutral state.

The positive and the negative results above are where our emotions and feelings are found. Depending on our response, the goal may be achieved or it may be totally unreachable.

The Avoidance Process

When we avoid a goal, we perceive it to be harmful. Anything that we perceive as negative is considered "non-approachable." So, the Avoidance Process involves two opposing sides that can lead to the following results:

If we do poorly, we experience fear and anxiety.

If we do well, we experience relief and calmness.

If we do it just right, we are in a neutral state.

In the same way, our emotional and feelings result from successfully avoiding something or not.

The relationships presented above lead us to understand where our emotions and feelings are functional as seen below:

The closer we are to the goal we intend to approach, the more joyous our emotions become and the happier we feel.

The farther we are from a goal we intend to approach, the more depressed our emotions become and the sadder we feel.

If we encounter an obstacle as we begin to approach our goal, the more attentive we become and the more motivated we feel to pursue it.

If we encounter an obstacle when we are nearing our goal, our emotions will become angrier and we will feel frustrated.

If we are farther from the goal we do not wish to pursue, the more relaxed our emotions will become and the more relieved we feel.

If we are closer to the goal we do not wish to pursue, the more fearful our emotions are and the more anxious we feel.

If we are closer to the goal we do not wish to pursue and something happens to get us out of it, the more surprised our emotions will be and the more relief we feel.

If we are far from the goal we do not wish to pursue and manage to get out of it even without doing anything, our emotions might cause us disgust and we might feel guilty.

If you follow the patterns above, the first set of behavior mentioned in each item is an emotion while the latter is a feeling. The same applies to what we do every day. This is to say that our feelings are a result of our emotions because our emotions are reactions to our environment. So how do we use this knowledge in order for us to keep on going for the goals we have in our lives?

How to Develop Emotional Awareness and Reach Your Goals

Understand the concept of emotional intelligence. Emotional intelligence is not the same as the concept of I.Q., but the same principle applies when people say that you have a high level of E.Q. That simply means you're better at relating to other people, you're better at managing your emotions, and you're better at using your emotions to achieve your goals. So, under this step, it pays to understand four concepts:

Self-awareness. You will never be able to understand others if you fail to understand yourself. Self-awareness in this context means understanding the triggers of certain emotions. Why do you experience such an emotion? What cues do you get from the environment? How do you recognize it?

Self-management. Recognizing and understanding your emotions is not enough if you don't know how to manage them. Managing your own emotions requires a certain degree of sacrifice and compromise that does not lead to feelings of frustration and dissatisfaction.

Social awareness. You can become aware of other people's emotions if you're good at recognizing your own. Social awareness entails a degree of understanding of your current environment and understanding the reason of other people's emotions. Without this level of understanding, you will never be able to find reason in other people's emotions.

Relationship management. This is the part where you relate to other people effectively in any social context and regardless of other people's behaviour, social status, race, etc.

Developing emotional awareness is important in propelling you to the achievement of your goals. Take the following steps in order to bring you closer into touch with your emotions.

Learn how to manage negative emotions. Positive emotions are pretty good to entertain because these make us feel better but negative emotions come off as a challenge. Seeking self-destructive ways to manage negative emotions leads to negative feelings, so learn about proactive ways to manage negative emotions so you can keep yourself in check.

Be agreeable and open minded. If you are the type of person who does not yield, this is the right time for you to start recognizing that each individual possesses a different idea. It is common for conflict to arise in any setting. Learn to be agreeable while keeping an eye on your goal. It is fine to be expressive but remember that your goal is there waiting.

Be empathetic. Empathy is a skill. Unfortunately, it's a skill that many do not have. To be able to empathize means to be able to walk in someone else's shoes whilst recognizing that the pair of shoes is not yours. Empathy can lead you closer to your goal if you learn how to relate to other people and if you understand how some of them are instrumental in goal achievement. If you make enemies out of spite, your goal will stay as it is forever.

Be critical. In fact, be critically positive. Keeping your emotions in a positive light might be difficult nowadays because we have a lot of things to think about. But you can start by analysing a given situation and acting on it in a rational manner. Notice how rational decisions cause minor impact when it comes to negative emotions. In most cases, they yield positive feelings all because you decided based on what is best.

Be optimistic. Maintaining a positive attitude is necessary if you are to maintain positive emotions. A positive attitude rarely leads to negative emotions. If you stay positive about reaching your goal, you are apt to survive the obstacles that may come. The same is true for those goals that you are trying to get away from.

Never avoid your emotions. People sometimes deny what they really feel. They even lie about it. Beware; lying leads to feelings of guilt so it compounds the amount of negative emotion you feel. Instead, recognize your current emotional state and acknowledge the feeling that goes with it. Plus, avoiding your emotions causes you to lose what you invested in your goal, it damages your relationships, and it is exhausting.

In our lives, we always have a choice. Our choices won't always be right, but they do not have to necessarily take us away from our goals. We always have a chance to start over. By keeping our emotions in check, we avoid experiencing undesirable feelings.

Is Emotional Intelligence Innate or Acquired?

Human characteristics that are innate are those which one is born with and from which instinctual responses are derived. A debate exists as to whether emotional intelligence is in-born and is part of a person's personality, or whether it can be acquired in adulthood even when one did not previously have it.

The term personality is used in psychology to refer to an individual's thoughts, emotions, behaviors and attitudes that are unique to that person. Emotions especially, are a core aspect of the subject of this book. For example, some people are by nature happy, talkative and full of energy while others can be described as having a steady, calm and reliable disposition. This is to mean that personality influences introversion and extroversion tendencies in people.

The reason why the subject of personality is of importance here is due to the fact that it is in-born or innate. Although we can improve on our personalities, the changes incurred will be very slight and will tend not to vary much from whom we innately are. Emotional intelligence on the other hand may involve the application of already present natural abilities into practical everyday situations, such as in exercising sound judgment based on clear thinking patterns.

Whereas two people may share common tendencies in reference to their personalities, the manner in which they apply themselves to real life situations will tend to be very different. For example, of two individuals with a melancholic personality, one may possess very high levels of personal motivation and ambition while the other one may not.

If as a manager you are seeking to employ someone as a salesperson, conducting a personality test will not be sufficient although it may show that the person is talkative and friendly enough to make contacts and sales. There would be need to know how a person would come under the pressure that comes with deadlines, and that they will persist in the face of insurmountable challenges and work-related disappointments. A test of their emotional intelligence would equip you with that kind of information.

An employee may have a very pleasant and 'fun' personality but that does not necessarily equate to being a success at the workplace. Employees that have high levels of emotional intelligence will be able to manage and control negative impulses that stem from their personalities in such a way as to bring themselves work related success.

Some studies claim that human beings are to a certain degree born with a measure of emotional intelligence, which they term as 'innate emotional intelligence'. They point to an infant's ability for emotional sensitivity, as well the potential they have to retain and later recall all the emotional information that they are taking in from their environments during infancy. This information later forms the core of an individual's emotional intelligence.

An infant emotionally learns over time to sense when its mother is angry because they associate some of her repetitive reactions to anger. As they grow, this stored information forms the basis from which they are able to sense other people's feelings. This so called 'innate intelligence' can be continually developed or damaged through life experiences.

It is very possible for an infant to start life with some degree of emotional intelligence and then unlearn it by imitating unhealthy emotional tendencies from his caregivers. Unhealthy environments of abuse and neglect can also contribute to this unlearning process. Similarly, some infants may show low levels of emotional sensitivity but with the right emotional nurturing, end up scoring very high as emotionally intelligent adults.

Chapter 12 Keep A Conversation Going

Good social skills hinge on being able to relate and talk to others in a normal fashion. They can also mean the difference between superfluous small talk and warm, meaningful connections. If you want more people to like you, you must learn how to talk to people in a likable way.

The main component to great conversation is empathetic listening. You may be a great listener, but how do you show it? The answer is simply that by being obvious about your empathetic listening, you will excite the other person, proving that you care about what he or she has to say. However, to be an empathetic listener, you must prove that you are listening.

While someone talks, look directly at the person and/or nod and interject with the occasional affirmative motion. When the person pauses, you may mention something directly related to what he or she is saying. Conversely, changing the subject, interrupting, staring into space, and appearing impatient for your turn to talk are all good ways to alienate the talker and ruin the conversation. You want to appear interested by making eye contact and by practicing reflective listening.

Reflective listening refers to the method of repeating back what someone says, showing them that you really did hear what they just said. You may repeat things back verbatim, or, you may rephrase them. Similarly, you may also come back with a reply that proves you were paying attention and are absorbing what the person is saying.

There are different kinds of conversationalists. For example, some just talk forever, never paying attention to social cues causing them to bore and drive other people away. Then, there are wallflowers who don't talk to anyone as they carefully observe their surroundings. Finally, there are confident interactors who enjoy talking to others and listening to their stories with genuine interest3. You can see which of the three is the most likable. You want to aim for confident interaction at all times when relating to others.

If you are a shy person, injecting yourself into a conversation can pose a challenge. You may feel inclined to just sit back and listen. While this is great (because listening is the most important foundation of good conversation), you are lacking the other component...talking about yourself. You must be willing to talk as well as listen if you want your conversations to go anywhere. Otherwise, you will bore people and come across as a silent wallflower with nothing to add to the conversation. If this happens, the only people who will talk to you will be the blowhards who talk incessantly and don't know when to shut up. You can avoid these problems by having confident interactions.

The key here is to actually talk to the person you are conversing with. A conversation goes two ways, and you must do your part to keep it going. On top of listening, you should start speaking.

Don't just interrupt by blurting out whatever comes to mind or by attempting to change the subject constantly. It's best to actually find relevant topics to bring up.

A relevant topic may be based on what the other person starts talking about. If you want to give the other person control of the conversation, then you can just go along with what he or she talks about. This is a good way to start practicing conversation with people if you are shy.

However, you can also take charge of conversations and propose your own topics. Wait for the other person to stop talking and then bring up a new topic. Possibly find topics that are somehow related to the original one proposed by the other person so that there is logical flow to the conversation.

Starting a conversation first gives you more control of the interaction and allows you to make a solid impression. You can start talking to someone and find ways to relate. Tip: keep mentioning topics until you find one that takes off.

The most relevant topic is one that can bond you and your conversation partner. Finding topics that actually interest both of you is a good way to pass the time without causing boredom or frustration. You will want to find things that you can relate to your conversation partner on, and the more you find in common, the more you will like each other. Briefly introduce yourself and talk about what you enjoy and see if your conversation partner resonates with anything you say.

Asking questions that lead to a person talking about themselves is another way to start a good conversation. Keep the focus on your conversation partner by asking him/her questions about themselves. Ask what he/she likes and for more details about his/her job. Then, if he/she mentions any topic, you should ask them to expand on it. People love to talk about themselves, so this can really encourage a person to open up and like you.

Similarly, you may inadvertently repel conversation and relationships with negativity. For instance, if someone mentions fly fishing and you say, "I hate fly fishing," you are creating a negative factor which can halt the bonding experience. It is far better to stay positive and say something like, "I have never tried fly fishing" or, "I'm not much of a fishing person, to be honest, but I do love being outdoors." Both examples dangle the possibility of still finding something in common in front of your conversation partner, even if you don't enjoy the particular hobby of fly fishing.

It has been found that people who share more and act more intimate or familiar right off the bat tend to make a better impression and make more friends. Therefore, you can actually enjoy more conversational success by acting more familiar with people you have just met. This applies to the warmth factor mentioned earlier. You may feel that this is wrong and that asking personal questions is rude, but people will actually open up to you more if you do.

This idea was proven by an interesting experiment where people were divided into two groups where members were assigned random partners. In one group, the pairs were told to exchange small talk; the other group was told to ask very personal questions from a list. All participants rated how much they liked each other before the experiment and after. The group who exchanged personal questions liked each other the most at the study's end. This is because they were actually able to form a bond and get to know each other.

Naturally, this does not mean that you should ask offensive or upsetting questions, nor will you want to ask someone about his/her religious or political affiliations as this can invite controversy and unpleasantness. Instead, ask personal questions that people might enjoy answering. Your goal is to get someone to divulge information to you so that you can find common ground over which to bond.

You might start conversations with refreshing personal questions that most people don't ask. For example, you might ask someone what he/she would do if they were to find out that they have one day left to live, or what his/her dream job was when he/she was still a kid. You might also consider asking someone about the best book he/she ever read or the most vivid dream he/she ever had. Because questions are not your typical, run of the mill conversation starters, they will intrigue and interest your conversation partner and make for quite dynamic conversation.

Another key to good conversation is to pay careful attention to the ebb and flow of the conversation. If a person starts to withdraw or look bored, don't take it personally. Instead, take it as a sign that you should change the subject. Similarly, if a person starts to get upset, you should definitely change the subject. Consider how to soothe and reassure a person who is not enjoying the topic. Be sure to acknowledge a person's feelings by saying, "I can see this is really important to you" or, "I can see that this upsets you a lot." This kind of emotional recognition makes a person feel validated. Validation is key to being liked.

You are not responsible for how someone feels, but if you want to have good conversation, you should try to keep things pleasant and light. No one really wants to talk about heavy topics, especially if they don't know you well.

Confident interaction involves showing that you are invested and interested. You must listen and you must speak. Maintaining the flow of conversation by going back and forth on relevant topics is the basis of the social skill of good conversation.

Chapter 13 Primal Leadership

Leadership comes in many different forms. We see leaders in politics, the military, and business. At its core, leadership means devising a plan to guide a team to victory. It involves establishing direction, constructing and sharing a clear vision, and inspiring others to join in the quest. Leadership always requires efficient management skills.

Constructing a Vision

A vision is more than just the picture that an individual has in his or her mind to depict success. It provides a finish line of sorts, that indicates the achievement of set goals. A vision must be realistic, but it's also utilized to inspire others and convince them that the goal is worthwhile. It sets the tone and makes priorities clear for anyone involved. A vision means that you're not quite satisfied with the status quo; you're proactively looking ahead.

It's a leader's job to make his or her vision fascinating, appealing, and convincing. The goal is to compel others by having them embrace your vision. As a leader, you'll inspire people by supplying them with a vivid picture of how the future will look once your objectives have been met. It's important to appeal to people in a way that makes your vision relatable to them.

Inspiration and Motivation

A vision is the essential start, but it will only get you so far. The next step in leadership is inspiring and motivating a team of people to work together to achieve a common goal: actualizing your vision.

Just as it gets challenging to motivate yourself once the novelty has worn off, motivating others also gets difficult over time. Enthusiasm fades. An effective leader anticipates this, and diligently works to continue the encouragement throughout the duration of the project. You'll need to continue to find ways to connect with your team, keep your vision at the forefront of their minds, and inspire them to keep pushing.

You can appeal to people's motivation in different ways. Efficient and effective leaders utilize both intrinsic and extrinsic motivators. For example, take a look at the following chain reaction:

hard work ➡ *positive results* ➡ *re*

Hard work yields positive results, which then produce a reward. This mentality appeal to team members' internal motivation (wanting to do a good job) and external motivation (wanting a reward).

Leaders often have power of some sort. For example, you might be in a position to issue paychecks or assign personnel changes. A good leader doesn't rely too heavily on these things when he or she is working to motivate others.

Management of the Vision

Part of your leadership role obviously entails management, but you're not merely managing people. For a goal to be successfully achieved, actualizing the vision requires work, and it needs to be managed. In order to achieve this, specific goals need to be set.

Any member of a team that is working on delivering your vision will need clear performance goals. These goals must correlate to your vision. You must also efficiently manage any change that is necessary, so that things run smoothly for everyone involved.

Coaching and Teamwork

As a leader, you're the coach of your team. Your job is not just to supervise; rather, you must make sure that everyone is equipped with the skills and strategies that are needed to fulfill your vision. A team dynamic means that development and training are key. Ensuring that all team members are fully capable happens through coaching, assessment, and feedback.

A leader always looks for leadership potential in members of his or her team. If you develop these skills in-house, you're creating sustainability, and the success of your team will continue into the future.

Leadership Skills

Leaders should always concern themselves with building the necessary competencies to be successful. There are numerous valuable skills involved in leadership, let's explore six of them.

1. Emotional intelligence is, as we know, to be in tune with your emotions and the emotions of others. A leader must be able to accurately read emotional situations and communicate with other people in a way that incorporates emotions. Building emotional intelligence involves practice. First, you can practice appropriately expressing and regulating your own emotions. You can also practice evaluating others' nonverbal communication. It's also important to expose yourself to different people and social environments so that you can practice engaging others and developing your perception. Put your listening skills to use and hone your communication abilities. Look at situations from the perspective of others.

2. *Conflict management skills are absolutely essential for a leader. When others are in disagreement, a leader can be called upon to mediate. An effective leader is able to successfully resolve these conflicts. It's also essential that you're able to resolve (or, better yet, avoid) your own conflicts. It's important to be able to generate solutions that are either a compromise or a win-win cooperation.*

3. *Decision making is a skill that is essential for a leader. It entails making good choices and also leading the process of making good choices. A successful leader knows when it's an appropriate time to make a decision. Additionally, he or she knows when to consult others or hand the responsibility to someone else. The best way to practice effective decision making is to learn from your mistakes. It's helpful to keep a mental inventory of what was involved in decisions you've made in the past, and whether or not the outcome was a success.*

4. *A successful leader has fortitude. It's necessary to have courage when you're taking risks, even when they're based on reliable information. Having*

fortitude means that you're not afraid to stand up for what's right. Developing fortitude involves supporting your team and standing by your principles.

5. *Good judgment is necessary for successful leadership. When you're able to open your mind to others' perspectives and consider different points of view, you make prudent decisions. Practicing good judgment means that you ask questions, consider other people's opinions, and understand the scope of your actions.*

6. *Of course, a successful leader needs to be competent in his or her area of expertise. While this was once the most important trait of a leader, we now know that the best leader for a team might not be the one with the most technical knowledge. It is important, though, for a leader to build his or her industry expertise and realize that development is a long-term process. Successful leaders take every opportunity to learn as much as they can. This can happen through getting to know team members, studying the competition, and educating yourself.*

Chapter 14 Identify Your Purpose

One of the fastest ways to attain our goals and be at peace with ourselves is by learning how to find our passion and purpose in life. Without having a sense of purpose to guide you in the right direction, you might end up feeling unfulfilled even after achieving your goals.

Each one of us is born with a unique life purpose (no two people have the same one). Identifying and honoring this objective in our lives is perhaps the most critical action successful individuals take. It's essential to take out time from our busy lives to understand why we're here on earth, and then pursue it with enthusiasm and passion.

For some people, it's already clear what their purpose in life is, right from when they're born. All of us were created with a set of talents, and while some of us quickly discover what they are on time and utilize these skills, a few others need to develop them through constant practice and determination.

Individuals born with natural talents end up honing them over time and ultimately turn the skills into something they're passionate about and use to achieve their dreams. For some, it takes hard work even to figure out if we're good at anything, so we end up giving up and doing what others are doing so we wouldn't feel left out. When you choose to do what you're not passionate about, you'll eventually start to notice life how your life is lacking a deeper meaning to it.

Explore the Things that Come Naturally to You

We're all born with a purpose that we have to discover during the process of our lives. It's not something you have to fake since it's already there; all that's required for you is to discover it. You need to uncover what your purpose is to build the life you want.

One of the easiest ways to figuring it out is to think about what you love doing or what comes effortlessly to you. Whatever your purpose is, it should feel natural – not forced. Work might be required to hone your skills after discovering them, but suffering isn't always necessary. If you're struggling and suffering to keep up with something you assumed was your purpose in life, then the chances are you're probably in the wrong field.

Sometimes the process is as simple as following what your heart tells you. A lot of people fail to realize that we all have an inner guidance system inside of us that helps us get to various points in our lives. You could think of it as an internal GPS of sorts which guides us through multiple aspects in our lives.

With every image you visualize while trying to realize your dreams, you're "Inputting" the particular destination you need to reach at a specific time. And each time you express your preference of something over the other, you're unconsciously stating an intention.

In most cases, the things that bring you the most amounts of joy and pleasure are aligned with your life's purpose even without knowing it.

Doing what you love increases your productivity levels

You'll notice that when you're doing what you enjoy and love you're more engaged and devoted to the exercise. You'll be motivated and excited to complete various tasks assigned to you by your boss or other people; this translates to an increase in productivity.

Individuals that genuinely love their jobs never feel tired of doing it. They remain motivated because their job doesn't feel like a chore to them. Focus on doing the things that drive you positively to avoid getting bored with your life. Passion differentiates good work from great ones.

Just by looking at your work, any sane person with a keen eye can tell if it was something you were passionate about or not. It all lies in your attention to details or not. Not only will the work you're excited about having premium quality, but it'll also have an emotional value attached to it.

Steps to Identify your Purpose

- First of all, understand what the term means

While there are many definitions of "Life Purpose" the main thing to note is that to identify it is to make an in-depth review of everything you've ever done in your life that brought meaning and fulfillment to it. Whatever you come to terms with needs to be simple and straightforward; it shouldn't be overcomplicated.

Your life's purpose could be to bring order and chaos to the lives of those around you, help others achieve their goals, or use your talents to bring change to the world. To begin identifying what it is, try connecting the dots from your childhood up to the point you are now and discover who you've always been and the impact you've made on people's lives.

- Honor what you love doing and slowly start separating yourself from the things that drain and exhausts you

The chances are that you won't be able to feel or honor your purpose in life if you're always tied down with activities that you dislike, or people you don't admire or respect. You'll find out that when you separate yourself from demoralizing situations and focus on things that motivate you to do better, that your sense of self-worth would begin to improve. Finding our life's purpose is only possible when we take action and honor our needs and values. The key here is to start behaving like you're worthy of having one in the first place and begin saying no to work and activities that you despise.

- Identify new ways you'd like to be of help to others

It could be through your hobbies, work, or volunteering for a cause that means a lot to you and others. For most individuals who focus on being of service to the people around them, they all agree that the act of helping out makes them feel alive and useful. It makes them feel like they're part of something greater than themselves.

You are your life's purpose because it shows in how you live, interact with others, support growth and positivity around you, and how you use your natural talents to add to the lives of others.

If you're still unsure of what your purpose is or how to discover it, just start with recognizing a new way to do something that not only gives you a sense of achievement but also fills you with joy as you're doing it.

Chapter 15 How To Deal With Negative Emotions In People

We are human beings, and therefore the emotional aspect of being human beings will always affect how we live. At any point in our lives, there are emotions that we have to deal with. We can choose to laugh or cry at whatever is happening in our lives. Unfortunately, negative emotions are the hardest to deal with. At times negative feelings overwhelm us to the point where we think of giving up. Learning how to control negative emotions will guarantee that we surround our lives with positivity. In spite of the things that we cannot control, we should be able to manage how we feel about them. Ultimately, this will have an impact on how we perceive our lives.

So, how do you control negative emotions from breaking you?

Eliminate Negative Thoughts

Managing negative emotions begins by eliminative negative thoughts. Negativity will always pull you down. You will always feel as though you woke up on the wrong side of your bed. Sadly, these feelings will also prevent you from seeing the good side of life. You will never see past obstacles that are stopping you from reaching your goals. Therefore, it is vital that you learn how to eliminate negative thoughts in your everyday life.

There are practical ways in which you could stop negative thoughts from affecting how you perceive things.

Talk to Your Negative Thoughts

The best way of dealing with your negative thoughts is not by avoiding them. Often, what you resist will persist. Therefore, it is essential that you become aware of these negative thoughts before anything else. How are you feeling? Are you tired, stressed, or frustrated? First, recognize your negative thoughts. To deal with them, embrace the idea of talking to these thoughts. This could be in the form of affirmations which remind you of the presence of the negative thoughts, but you are choosing not to believe in them. Ideally, affirming to yourself that you are in control will bestow you with the mind control you need to see past your challenges.

ASSOCIATE WITH POSITIVE PEOPLE

Additionally, getting rid of negative feelings requires that you associate yourself with like-minded people. If you are trying to transform your life, find someone who is already in the position you wish to be in. Make friends and maintain your friendship. Identifying yourself with people who have a direction in life will also give you a sense of direction. You will begin to see the positive side of living. Therefore, you will refrain from thinking negatively as most of your friends focus on the bright side. With regards to emotional intelligence, find someone who is better than you. Learn from them on how to live an optimistic life. Ultimately, you will quash negative thoughts in your mind.

LOWER YOUR EXPECTATIONS

Indeed, it is good to live an optimistic life. Nevertheless, this doesn't mean that you should have high expectations. Expecting things to be perfect will simply prevent you from being happy. Your vision of success should be closely tied to reality. Knowing that you will succeed in the long run will give you a reason to be patient for the best results. In turn, you will never rob yourself of true happiness that you should be enjoying now.

CREATE A POSITIVE MORNING ROUTINE

Psychologists will argue that controlling your thinking will help you control your life [2]. There is some truth to this. What you think about mostly, is what you will eventually become. So, start your day on a high note by encouraging yourself. This eliminates negative feelings and boosts your energy throughout the day.

Overcome Stress and Anxiety

Negative emotions will often lead to feeling stressed out and anxious. To manage negative feelings from arising through stress and anxiety, the following tips should help you.

EXERCISE REGULARLY

Regular exercise will help you deal with stress in many ways. The idea of pushing your body to the limits through exercise can really help boost your mental health. Research also shows that people who engage in physical activities frequently will lower their chances of feeling anxious [3]. There are several reasons which could help in explaining this.

First, exercising lowers stress hormones in your body. Equally, regular exercise releases endorphins. These are chemicals responsible for enhancing your moods. Your sleep quality will also be improved through engaging in physical activities. The best part is that regular exercise will help you feel confident about yourself and your abilities. Inviting these good feelings to your life will definitely aid in eliminating negative vibe in your life.

CHECK YOUR DIET

Exercising routinely should be complemented by eating the right foods. The mere fact that you should overcome stress and anxiety implies that you ought to stay away from stress and anxiety triggers. Alcohol and caffeine, for example are known to increase the likelihood of feeling anxious [4]. Your caffeine intake should be avoided as this will make you feel nervous or increase your irritability. It is important to note that stopping your caffeine intake immediately will have negative withdrawal symptoms. Therefore, it is recommended that you should reduce your intake gradually.

IT SHALL PASS

Sometimes it is good to remind yourself that you are not the only individual going through stress in your life. In fact, some are going through harder situations. So, you need to brace yourself and keep your head up. Overcoming negative feelings that come with stress could be aided by having the mentality that the situation shall pass. The negative feeling that you are experiencing will pass. The important thing you need to bear in mind is that you are trying to make yourself stronger by believing that you can overcome the situation.

Overcome Social Anxiety and Shyness

Negative feelings can also be handled through the idea of overcoming social anxiety and shyness. The idea of being anxious when conversing with other people will invite negative feelings about yourself. You will never feel confident to approach people and express yourself. People will think that you are shy. From you end, you will suffer as you will always hide in your cocoon with no friends to help you out. Below are strategies which will help you conquer social anxiety and shyness in your life.

ADMIT THE FEAR

The first thing that you need to do is to admit that there is fear within you. Accepting the fact that you have that fear is an extremely important first step in overcoming your problems. You cannot deal with something or a condition without identifying it. The importance of acknowledging the problem you are facing helps in realizing that you are better than what you think. It gives you a reason of seeing past your fears or shyness.

ENGAGE ACTIVELY

Fighting your shyness by engaging actively is an approach which could also work. If there is someone you like, approach them and be frank about it. Sure, you will be rejected a few times, but you will realize that there is nothing to fear. After all, there is no one who will be harmed from your rejection. You cannot expect everyone around you to like you. So, anticipate that there will be a few rejections you will have to deal with. Adopting this mentality gives you courage to overcome social anxiety. There is nothing to be afraid of and that there is no harm in trying.

Get Out of Your Comfort Zone

Being shy will drive you to avoid people at all cost. Reserved people will prefer to be left alone in their own worlds. However, you need to challenge yourself. Engage in activities regardless of whether they make you anxious. Participate in social games as this is what will gradually boost your confidence levels. Don't allow your fear to get the best of you. Challenge yourself by facing your fears head on. It might be a daunting task from the word go, but eventually, you will rip the fruits.

Body Language

Your body language will also need transformation if you wish to overcome your anxiety. This will not come easily as you will have to practice regularly through the small conversations you enter into. When talking to people, try to make eye contact. Speak loudly for people to hear you clearly. If possible, give hugs and shake hands. Working on your body language will boost your confidence in great ways.

From the information discussed in this section, dealing with negative emotions is not as challenging as you might have assumed. It all boils down to what you think about. As part of making sure that you live a productive life, always ensure that you associate yourself with the right people. The influence you get from them will have a huge impact on your life. Similarly, you need to find a way out of stressful situations. Go to the gym and workout. Give your body and opportunity of releasing endorphins to help you feel good. Inviting positive vibes your way is an ideal way of banishing negative feelings.

Conclusion

In conclusion, social skills are very important. Whether the language and cultures are different, but social skills are very similar everywhere.

Another thing is understanding empathy and how it is used. Empathy is the act of placing oneself in other people's shoes. When talking to people, someone should try and understand others and their issues. This is where listening comes in. The importance of listening is that one cannot feel what others feel if you do not even listen to them. Putting yourself out there for others to rely on your support is important in being empathetic. Empathy is just a virtue that people should ignore, but everyone should embrace it.

Communication also involves the aspect of cognition. Cognition is the mental activities. Communication does not just happen without any thinking through. Thinking is essential during communication. One has to think of what others think and also what they feel. One has to consider other opinions and make sure to take them into consideration at any time. The way one takes a conversation in mind determines how the conversation will be or the final result. A conversation is supposed to be thought through since it is not a joke except while with friends, but that too should be taken seriously.

Also, emotions are key in terms of communication. One should know how emotions are applied in the world of communication. Emotions help to guide communication between people. Without understanding emotions, then it is going to be hard to read in between the lines of each communication. Without an understanding of emotions, then one can hardly understand things like jokes or even sarcasm. This is an important aspect of communication which is used every day and at any time. So, emotions are very important whether happy, sad or even mad. Everyone should work on their emotional radar for proper and better communication.

There also applications of communication. This refers to the uses of communication in our daily humanly lives. These applications are at work, school, and also at home. Communication varies with every place and time. It is a times official, and other times it is not at all official. Official language comes in at work and sometimes at school. Work the language is official but outside it is different all in all. In school, it depends on who you are talking to since student to student conversation is very informal while with the teachers, it is very formal. The family or at home the means of communication is formal.

To finish up this book gives you the see-through of how communication is important. It also shows that communication does not occur for a person only. One then should learn to relate with others even if they are going to communicate with other people. Language has also been seen to be crucial in terms of communication. It is also important to know the emotions of a person, especially during any sort of communication.